Problem-based Learning in a Health Sciences Curriculum

Problem-based learning is an approach which places the student at the centre of the learning process and is aimed at integrating learning with practice. In this book, the contributors draw on their experience of designing and implementing a course for nurse education in Australia to present effective strategies for those considering adopting the approach or adapting it to their own curricular needs. The book identifies the advantages of such a method of learning in nursing and indicates how these might be extended to allied health disciplines, education and distance education.

Each chapter addresses a particular aspect of problem-based learning, such as developing learning packages in Chapters 1 and 2, looking at possible future questions for problem-based learning and considering the necessary conditions for the development and maintenance of such a course. Other chapters discuss the integration of various types of knowledge and evaluation and in Chapter 10 particular emphasis is put on guidance for adapting the course to use within a more traditional curriculum. All the chapters are presented from a very practical perspective with detailed examples.

Problem-based Learning in a Health Sciences Curriculum is based on the contributors' first-hand experience of setting up a problem-based course and the evaluation and comments from students quoted in the book illustrate their enthusiastic response to this type of learning. It   who want to explore and extend their teaching met social workers, occupational therapists and psychc

Christine Alavi is a nurse and psychologist. She the School of Nursing at Griffith University, Queensland, Australia.

Problem-based Learning in a Health Sciences Curriculum

Edited by Christine Alavi

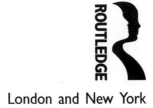

London and New York

First published 1995
by Routledge
11 New Fetter Lane, London EC4P 4EE

Simultaneously published in the USA and Canada
by Routledge
29 West 35th Street, New York, NY 10001

Typeset in Times by
Florencetype Ltd, Stoodleigh, Devon
Printed and bound in Great Britain by
Clays Ltd, St Ives PLC

British Library Cataloguing in Publication Data
A catalogue record for this book is available from
the British Library

Library of Congress Cataloguing in Publication Data
A catalogue record for this book has been requested

ISBN 0–415–11207–9 (hbk)
ISBN 0–415–11208–7 (pbk)

To all the graduates of 1993

Vivien Adams, Sue Alexander, Caroline Allison, Simone Andrews, Susan Appleby, Anika Austin, Sonia Barjasic, Josie Barnes, Elvira Barrios, Elizabeth Bergstrum, Jenny Berrell, Mandy Boswell, Janette Boyce, Wynita Brennan, Fiona Brett, Jennifer Bryant, Jenny Burton, Sandra Castle, Julie Chan-Versluis, Ria Cirson, Renea Collins, Phoebe Collins, Justine Coulson, David Crofts, Gabrielle Curtain, Rosina Daley, Lisa Dawson, Tanya Degney, Nikki Devencorn, Gerri Doogan, Jenny Doolan, Kerri Dooley, Anne Duncan, Tyrone Dungey, Lyn Dunham, Christine Durant, Karen Eastman, Tracey Eleison, Keith Elsden, Yvonne Eriksen, Liz Fountain, Margie Fox-Fryer, Karen Gallagher, Marie Gallibu, Pierette Garner, Renata Geary, Kelly Gifford, Liz Grant, Agnes Gutugutuwai, Rikki Hall, Lisa Hay, Damien Hayes, Pam Haynes, Karen Herbert, Bonnie Houston, Karen Jeynes, Sharon Johnson, Kerri Jones, Melissa Jones, Vicki Jurgevics, Nicola Kennedy, Monika Kilpatrick, Tony King, Astrid Klemmt, Carmela La Pila, Joanne Ladewig, Colin Larwood, Samantha Lee, Robyn Lindsay, Janine Lindsay, Megan Long, Natalie Luxton, Desaree Martinez, Patricia McCabe, Brigid McCarthy, Betty McDonald, Michelle McDonnell, Annemaria McGinn, Fran McKindley, Antoinette McLeod, Sally McPherson, Gillian Melksham, Julie Miller, Sonya Miru, Kim Mitchell, Jeremy Monk, Sarah Moreny, Clare Murray, Clare Nally, Jodi Nimmo, Megan O'Sullivan, Carolina Orellana, Matthew Parnaby, Ann Parnell, Mandy Parravicini, Linda Pforr, Fiona Pullar, Maree Richards, Anthony Rietberg, Sarah Ross, Nicole Roxburgh, Esther Schrijver, Phillip Schwarz, Nadine Smith, Allan Smith, Helen Squires, Leanne Stark, Deborah Stevens, Linda Stevenson, Leisha Stoneley, Michele Stubbs, Jillian Sutton, Sara Thompson, Jocelyn Toohill, Cathryn Vermeer, Annette Vermulm, Richard Walker, Angela Warland, Kerry Watson, Melinda Waugh, Heather Wells, Ingrid Werner, Terri White, Bern White, Marie Williams, Kirsty Williams, Kerryn Williams, Rebecca Young, Anneleis Zeissink.

Contents

Contents

Illustrations

Tables

Acknowledgements

This book comes from our development of a problem-based programme at Griffith University, Brisbane, Queensland. Our thanks go to many people. From the original planning group we particularly acknowledge Betty Anderson and Arthur Brownlea. Penny Little and Greg Ryan were unfailingly supportive and helpful. Clinical agencies too numerous to mention generously contributed clinical material. The participating students have shared our learning with us. Those who supported the programme – particularly Lyn Armit, Barry Cliff, Marie Crowe, Anne Donovan, Anne Fairbairn, Jenny Morris, Debbie Osborne, Gerard Pulle, Judy Wilkie and Kethia Wilson – thank you. The members of the Centre for the Advancement of Learning and Teaching were always available with guidance or just to listen.

John Frow was generous with his time and expertise.

Jenny Chan patiently and very good-humouredly typed the manuscript.

Most of all we thank each other. As co-authors we have each contributed to all the chapters of the book. The opportunity to work together in developing the programme and writing this book has been a pleasure and a privilege.

Introduction

What kind of curriculum will best help students to become competent professional practitioners? Every new course should start with an answer to this question, preferably an explicit answer. This book is developed around the answer taken in one new nursing degree course. You will discover why and how a course of study beginning with lectures was rejected and instead we had students start by examining the following scenario:

> Sonia Hepinstall is a student in your group. She has come from a small town 200 km away to start the problem-based nursing course. She has always wanted to be a nurse and is particularly drawn to emergency department nursing. Her aunt, a registered nurse who has worked in a busy metropolitan teaching hospital, has told her that university nursing courses are no good as they don't have enough 'hands-on' experience and that all you have to do is write assignments. Sonia wonders if she has made the right choice.

This example will be discussed in more detail later. However, in the wider context, an increasing number of health-care departments and schools in universities around the world are coming to see problem-based learning courses as the best answer to our opening question.

> *It's really just suited me to the ground. I think being able to go out and do your own research and get it by yourself for the group; it's a better way to learn, you're actually learning not just getting it thrown at you.*
>
> Peter, Year 1 student

But what is a 'problem-based learning course'? This question is especially important because problem-based learning is often confused with case-study approaches to learning, discovery learning and project-based learning. Sometimes even the most orthodox lecture-based courses are described by their practitioners as 'problem-based' on the grounds that they include an opportunity for students to solve textbook 'problems' during tutorials. In this view almost any course might be described in a similar way. A much clearer understanding of problem-based learning is needed if problem-based courses are to be designed and run effectively. Such an understanding has been developing over the past few decades as experience of this form of education has grown.

Problem-based learning can be described in many ways, but it is possible to see at least three common threads in all of them. First, there is a clear purpose in regard to an area of study, namely, to integrate practice and theory so as to produce sound understanding and action. Second, there is an educational process carefully considered and designed to achieve this purpose. Third, the process is itself content-specific and reflects the process which led to the generation of knowledge in the area of study in the first place. This third thread can be explained more fully along the following lines. A problem-based learning course is not a course in general problem-solving, but focuses specifically on content (or subject-matter) central to the area of study by requiring students to acquire important knowledge in the process of tackling problematic situations. In effect, by combining a problem-tackling process with the specific knowledge essential to dealing with the problem in question, problem-based learning reflects the real process of knowledge generation, regardless of whether the knowledge is 'pure' (generated by questions of pure curiosity) or 'applied' (generated by questions of practical importance). Problem-based learning is open to whatever considerations are relevant to dealing with a problematic situation; it makes no prior commitments to particular subjects or disciplines but is open to taking into account whatever will help deal with the problem. In this it reflects a significantly different conception of knowledge and understanding from conceptions which presuppose that knowledge is certain, on the basis of unshakeable foundations, and incorrigible and that it must be divided up in the ways typically represented in university departments. It posits a more tentative character to knowledge, possibly an evolutionary character, in contrast to a conception of knowledge as fixed eternally. It treats theory and practice as distinguishable rather than as categorically different, and therefore finds no difficulty in treating real problem-situations as central in the educational context.

The similarity between an original situation of knowledge acquisition in response to problems and a problem-based learning situation often leads to a misunderstanding of problem-based learning. It is sometimes thought that problem-based learning is wasteful of time and energy since it seems to be merely a process of re-inventing the wheel. This misunderstanding often arises because the difference between the original situation and the educational situation is overlooked. In a good problem-based learning course problems are judiciously selected, their presentation is thoroughly designed, and the way they are tackled by students is carefully facilitated – and, most importantly, the sequence of problems throughout the course as a whole must be equally thoroughly designed. A vital principle of problem-based course design is a requirement to reflect the actual problem situation as realistically and as fully as possible in the educational context, while structuring the presentation of the problem in such a way that effective learning by students can be achieved within the time available in the course. This may sound like an impossible balancing act, but examples of how it is achieved are contained in the chapters in this book. The effect, far from a wasteful re-inventing of the wheel, is effective learning by students not only of the necessary knowledge in the sense of content, but also of the process of acquiring important knowledge as necessary in new situations.

There is, in this, a kind of process of discovery by students. However, it needs to be clearly distinguished from discovery learning. A criticism of the latter was that it did tend in many cases to drop the learner in at the deep end with little guidance; too often this resulted in students floundering. Problem-based learning avoids this difficulty by the selection of problems appropriate to the educational purpose; by a structured presentation of the problems related to the level of under-standing of the students concerned and by facilitation, which is to say tutoring that helps students to think creatively, intelligently, critically and sensitively about the problem-situation in question. This guides them where necessary and in a non-didactic way to knowledge they may be in danger of overlooking in their investigations, and it ensures an effective balance between acquiring knowledge and using it and understanding it appropriately.

A lot of us were expecting them to be like a school teacher . . . it was a whole change of concept, they're not there to teach us but to help us learn.
Andrew, Year 1 student

The importance of the use of knowledge may suggest a similarity between problem-based learning and case-study learning, particularly as problems can be thought of as cases. Case-study approaches capture to some extent the reality of actual situations and they generate more active student learning than do lectures, but their didactic element detracts from the self-directed learning of problem-based courses where students make much fuller use of their existing knowledge in order to gain new knowledge and understanding. Examples described in the following chapters show both how students do this and how the course systematically tests students' understanding and use of the knowledge they have acquired. The question of the use of knowledge, and the possible similarity of projects and problems, is sometimes taken to indicate that project-based learning is the same as problem-based learning. Where the project is a problem, then of course there may be quite strong similarities, although other aspects of problem-based learning – such as well-structured facilitation – may be absent. In other cases, however, where the project is a theme or a general idea rather than a problem, the distance from problem-based learning increases.

Problem-based learning, then, may quite easily be mistaken for other approaches to learning which resemble it in several ways. None the less, it is distinctive. In appearance, particularly as regards the processes observable in problem-based tutorials, the distinctiveness can be quite striking to those more familiar with raked lecture theatres containing serried ranks of fixed seats with students taking notes from the lecturer. A problem-based course does not begin with a series of lectures; it begins with a problem-situation which the students have to begin to deal with in a problem-based tutorial. A belief in the necessity of lectures reflects an assumption that students must absorb certain quantities of information through lectures or lecture-like media (such as didactic teaching texts in distance education) before they will be in a position to think about a subject. In contrast, in a problem-based learning course students begin with a problem because they are assumed not to be entirely devoid of knowledge. They know enough to form an initial understanding of the problem, they can reflect on it, critically evaluate what they think they know about it and what they do not; they may have some idea of how and where they might find out what needs to be known in order to understand the problem more fully, and so on. All this will be rudimentary compared to what they will know and be able to do by the end of the course.

Typically, then, having been presented with a problem-situation, students will work co-operatively in small groups in coming to grips with the problem, in formulating it adequately, in identifying what they need to learn in order to deal with it and so on; there will be fewer contact sessions between staff and students, although these are likely to be of longer duration than the normal lecture; the curriculum will show no division into separate subjects; during contact sessions with staff there will be considerable interaction and intellectual activity among students; and outside contact sessions students will be learning in other ways from various resources (written texts, multi-media, expert persons, films and others).

In its modern form problem-based learning has been a distinctive method since the 1950s when Case Western Reserve University began developing a problem-based course in its medical faculty. Since then other notable examples of problem-based courses have appeared at such institutions as McMaster University in Canada, the University of Newcastle in Australia, the Rijksuniversiteit Limburg at Maastricht in the Netherlands, and in areas of study from the health professions to engineering, architecture, optometry, law, metallurgy and social work. An early example in nursing occurred at the University of Western Sydney at Macarthur, Australia; Griffith University, Australia, now has a fully integrated problem-based learning course, and many other schools of nursing, particularly in South East Asian countries, are adopting this form of education.

While these examples are quite recent, problem-based learning has arguably been in existence for a much longer period in more or less closely related forms. Projects as named components in curricula first appeared in 1908 in connection with agricultural courses in Massachusetts, and these may be regarded as an early form of problem-based learning. In medieval medical schools students learned by following the qualified practitioner on rounds and observing what was said and done. Perhaps the earliest example of a kind of problem-based learning is the description Plato gives in the *Meno* of Socrates presenting a slave boy with a geometrical problem and, by questioning, getting him to see the inadequacy of his original solution to the problem and to think through to a satisfactory solution. However, in its modern form, in the second half of the twentieth century, problem-based learning has been practised in a quite distinctive way.

Problem-based learning places the student at the centre of the learning process and emphasises co-operative learning. The role of the teacher changes so that she becomes a resource for the students, facilitating their learning rather than being merely a purveyor of information. This method of learning has many implications which range from curriculum design to staff development, from educating the profession of nursing to persuading the students that we are adamant in acknowledging that even as novices they come to the university with a great deal of useful and relevant knowledge.

We will discuss all of these issues in more detail in the chapters which follow, but as an introduction to problem-based learning let us look again at the learning stimulus material given at the beginning of the introduction. It was developed to orientate students to a problem-based course in nursing at Griffith University, and will exemplify the learning process used in the first week of such a course.

Students generally come to university with preconceived ideas about nursing, learning and assessment that they have gained from a variety of sources, such as school, the media, friends, relatives and from other personal experiences. These might include the idea that nurses work only with those who are ill; that learning is always directed by the teacher; and that assessment is individual and competitive. These notions are quickly challenged, initially through the following first block of learning stimulus material:

> *Sonia Hepinstall is a student in your group. She has come from a small town 200 km away to start the problem-based nursing course. She has always wanted to be a nurse and is particularly drawn to emergency department nursing. Her aunt, a registered nurse who has worked in a busy metropolitan teaching hospital, has told her that university nursing courses are no good as they don't have enough 'hands-on' experience and that all you have to do is write assignments. Sonia wonders if she has made the right choice.*

This material is supported by suggestions about how to use time; details about off-campus clinical experience associated with the package; a list of suggested and available resources; and references indicative of the concepts and issues related to this package.

The learning material above is deliberately constructed with triggers to initiate discussion on the nature of nursing; on problem-based learning; on assessment; on clinical experience within the course; on living away from home; and on learning within a university setting. The purpose of these triggers is to orientate students to the course and to confront their preconceived ideas.

The role of the teacher here is that of a facilitator of student learning. What this means is that students are guided to develop analytical enquiry skills in processing information. They are encouraged, in effect, to learn how to learn; to be active participants in their own learning rather than passive recipients of the teacher's expertise. To this end each facilitator works collaboratively with a group of students – perhaps 15–20 in number – meeting them on a regular basis to process the learning material.

> *We've been taught to question. We've sort of learned through our group process to question things, and I think when we get out there very few of us will not have the confidence to keep asking questions.*
>
> *Anna, Year 3 student*

By the end of the first two-hour tutorial of the week students will have identified issues about which they need to learn more, how they might organise themselves to do this, and what might be some of the resources available to them. In order for students to achieve this they will be guided by the facilitator to read the learning material and to identify, by means of discussion and using their own experiences, what problems Sonia might have. The facilitator might encourage students to share their own thoughts and feelings about coming to university, and might help students to draw parallels between Sonia's experience and their own. Through the techniques of questioning, reflecting students' comments, validating their experiences and encouraging their contributions, the facilitator demonstrates clearly how the students' input is valued, promoting an atmosphere in which students feel comfortable to speak and can begin to share responsibility for the functioning of the group. Here, as throughout the course, students are encouraged to see problems not simply in negative terms but rather as situations in need of improvement (SINIs), where clients are viewed as needing some action from students placed in the role of registered nurses. Thus, the situation Sonia needs to improve concerns her doubt: has she made the right choice?

This material is specifically designed to be ambiguous so that it allows students to explore a range of issues that might be contributing to Sonia's situation. Identified issues may include her concern that university courses might not have 'hands-on' experience; difficulties she might have encountered living away from home; a particular view of nursing (busy emergency-based nursing); uncertainty about assessment in a problem-based course (all you have to do is write assignments); and general uncertainty about the nature of learning. There may also be rather idiosyncratic issues which might be raised and which may be directly related to what the students are themselves experiencing, but at this stage no issues are dismissed as fanciful or not useful. In working through this process students are introduced to the generation of hypotheses, the beginnings of the clinical reasoning process which they will progressively develop throughout the course. Before the tutorial ends the facilitator prompts the students to organise themselves to discover how they might test these hypotheses in the following three-hour self-directed learning time and, given that they are a group of twenty students, to develop some effective strategies for doing this in order to maximise their learning.

In considering the hypotheses the facilitator helps the individuals in the group who might choose to explore issues alone, or in pairs or small groups, to identify where they might find the information they need, and how they might go about presenting their findings to the group at the one-hour situation-review tutorial later in the day.

There is usually a great deal of turbulence at this point, some students being angry that the 'teacher' does not give the answers, some students being a little confused about what is expected of them and others feeling excited at being able to investigate the learning issues they have identified.

When the students reconvene in their tutorial group later in the day to present their findings they bring back information gleaned from various sources which allows them to begin to test the hypotheses they generated earlier. As has been the case on other problem-based learning courses, we were surprised at the range of activities students undertook in this time. Some students use written texts as their main sources whilst others are more adventurous and might, for example, have spoken to the Health Department about nursing; might have interviewed someone in the university about assessment; might have interviewed Student Services about what support is available for students who are living away from home, or may have discussed nursing issues with registered nurses working in various settings. The information is shared in a variety of ways. Students may bring back posters, overhead transparencies which give information or videos, or they may choose to role-play their information. In the light of this the group together decides which hypotheses they can reject, which they can accept and those that require further information before any definitive decision to accept or reject can be made. In such a case hypotheses are held for further exploration.

> *One of the benefits of problem-based learning as opposed to lectures is that you can go off on tangents that make links, and even wild guesses as to why someone has a problem. In a lecture you only have the lecturer's point of view.*
>
> *Jane, Year 3 student*

In these early days the facilitator's main role is to encourage students' self-directedness and assist students to develop confidence in their enquiry skills. Such a role is crucial as it helps students form the basis for their forays into the analysis of increasingly complex situations in need of improvement as the course progresses.

Unanswered questions raised at this time form the stimulus for further enquiry. To some extent these questions can have been anticipated and appropriate fixed-resource sessions for the total student population planned, given the deliberate structuring of the learning material. A fixed-resource session is a period of time when the whole student group gathers to explore learning issues. They are helped in this by experts who make themselves available to answer student questions. In the first week the resource persons might include a librarian who could answer questions on the use of the library; a behavioural scientist who might answer questions and initiate exercises about communication and working in groups; a biological scientist who might talk about the integration of science learning in the nursing course; or a panel of nursing faculty who can answer questions on assessment, problem-based learning and clinical experience within the course.

The nursing laboratory is a regular feature of student experience in any nursing course. It provides a safe place for students to rehearse behaviours and psychomotor skills which they will need to perform in off-campus nursing contexts. A nursing laboratory planned as a fixed-resource session in the first week might give the students an opportunity to practise and evaluate their communication skills, to help them take part in an off-campus clinical activity where, in order to discover more about nursing, they can talk to nurses from various clinical areas about their roles and functions. The person who co-ordinates students' clinical learning could previously have arranged for nurses in child health, paediatrics, maternity, community health, various hospital wards and departments, mental health, occupational health and school health to have made time available to spend with a group of students.

The final tutorial of the week serves two purposes. It allows students to summarise and consolidate their learning during the week, enabling them to review the concepts and issues they identified. As well, a period of time is set aside for students and their facilitator to discuss and analyse the working of the group throughout the week. After this process students might be encouraged (some time could be allocated) to reflect on group experiences, writing their thoughts, feelings and experiences in a private journal.

Why use such a method of teaching-learning – a method which, during the early days of a course, is very labour intensive in the designing of appropriate learning packages and the gathering of resources; which means that tutorials of no more than twenty students are the primary way of processing information; which makes traditional lectures almost non-existent; and which involves a radical rethinking of the way a nursing course is developed, taught and experienced?

Our thinking went something like this. Because nursing is a practice-based profession it is important that the learning reflects a nursing focus so students encounter situations on-campus which mirror, and are directly derived from, those which they will meet in the clinical area. Since nurses also work in multidisciplinary teams which must function amicably and co-operatively, it will benefit students if they work in groups from the beginning of the nursing course. Such group work needs therefore to be valued; co-operative learning which uses a mix of group assessments with individual assessments convinces students that working together is an important component of their learning.

Our motivation for writing this book is, in part, to share some of the strategies we used in order to establish a problem-based course which intimately integrates learning from the sciences, arts, the law, ethics and nursing by structuring these knowledges in learning packages developed from real-life situations where nursing interventions are made. Such knowledges are reiterated in different client situations and with increasing complexity throughout the course. Many examples of such learning packages are given throughout the book. An integrated and reiterative problem-based course, while a more successful way for students to learn, is no more expensive in terms of either human or material resources than a more traditional approach.

Each of the following chapters will address a particular aspect of problem-based learning as it has been identified in the design of a Bachelor of Nursing course. (To give some indication of the generic nature of the course, different packages will be used to exemplify the information.) In this way it will become apparent how such a course is able to address client situations across the life span, those with high and low dependence, in primary, secondary and tertiary health-care settings, in general, psychiatric, palliative care, maternity, child and extended care contexts as well as in multicultural settings.

In the first chapter, we would like to give you the opportunity to participate in a problem-based learning package from beginning to end. This is followed by a chapter which will deal in detail with the construction of learning packages, beginning with a discussion of conceptual and curriculum issues. It will move on to elaborate the design of learning triggers, resource material and referencing, incorporating a discussion of the processes of identifying and gathering resources. It will highlight the varied ways in which packages can be constructed, the material derived and the packages evaluated.

A chapter addressing facilitation in this problem-based context follows, with the focus here on the challenge it presents for educators in a practice-based discipline like nursing. Issues of the differences from traditional teaching methods; locus of control; student-teacher dyad; group learning; characteristics of good facilitation; and the tailoring of facilitation to problem-based learning will be addressed, along with some discussion of evaluation of facilitation by self, students and peer methods.

Chapters 4, 5 and 6 will address the issues of integration of knowledges. Chapter 4 deals specifically with how the science-learning needs of the student can be addressed. Discussion will include how experts from various disciplines contribute to the development of, and teaching and assessment within, a problem-based learning nursing course.

The integration of student learning in the nursing laboratory is dealt with in the following chapter. Examples of innovative worksheets which permit students to progress at their own pace within the relatively safe nursing laboratory environment are provided as they mirror situations which students will meet in the clinical context. Integrating knowledge in the clinical area is discussed in Chapter 6, where research into students' experience of clinical practice is used to show which elements in the clinical setting students anticipate and find most difficult or challenging, and how a problem-based course using clinical facilitators helps students deal with these elements.

Chapter 7 deals with the importance of orientation and transition to the facilitator role for teachers who are discovering and developing problem-based learning. The chapter discusses staff selection, orientation, continuing education and support, and gives examples of strategies used to promote team building.

Assessment occupies a central position in any course, particularly from the student perspective, but within problem-based learning it forms an integral part of the learning process. This perspective is elaborated more fully in Chapter 8, where innovative assessment strategies include student, self, peer and facilitator assessment. Individual and group assessment items, and examples of both formative and summative assessment formats and their contribution to effective student learning, are described and discussed.

Chapter 9 discusses evaluation of problem-based learning. It considers the role of evaluation in the problem-based learning curriculum: how it can be used to aid curriculum and staff development, and how it can empower students.

Chapter 10 examines how aspects of problem-based learning can be introduced into more traditional programmes. The authors make suggestions about how such transitions may be approached.

In the final chapter the authors take a speculative look at possible futures and questions for problem-based learning, considering the necessary and sufficient conditions for the development and maintenance of such a course.

Chapter 1
Approaching problem-based learning

Marie Cooke and Christine Alavi

> *Holistic approach. Problem-based learning provides problem-solving experiences ... learning is enhanced in an environment that is conducive to the free exchange of questions and ideas and one in which the uniqueness of each learner is valued. This is why peer/self evaluation is important. Through problem-based learning the learner is able to enhance their knowledge/skill individually in order to function effectively as a nurse when facing different situations and problems as well as have the ability to work with other team members. Responsibility of the faculty is to facilitate an optimal learning environment.*
>
> *Sarah, student*

We invite you to approach problem-based learning through an experience similar to the one students encounter. Rather than explain the process by which students engage with the learning material, we would like to give you the opportunity to work through a block of learning material in a structured learning package entitled *Timothy Randall*.

> We will guide you through Block 1 and give you the opportunity to work through Block 2 of this package.

For those who do not wish to work through Block 2, further explanation of the whole learning process will follow in future chapters. If you choose to continue with this chapter you will probably identify issues which raise queries, and we would encourage you to jot down ideas or questions for further investigation. Let us proceed then by putting this material into context.

Students, in groups of approximately twenty, have come to the point of engaging with this learning package by working in Semester 1, through similarly structured learning packages which focus on the themes of health, wellness and culture. This package, *Timothy Randall*, is the second of three packages placed in Semester 2, Year 1. All three packages have the theme of loss, and all contain core concepts

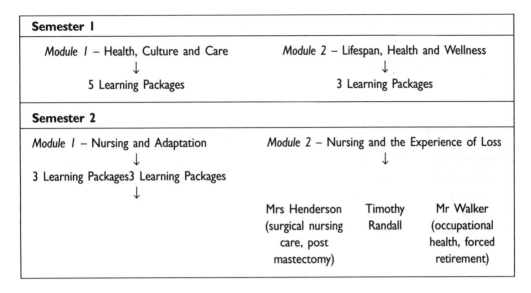

Figure 1.1: Organisation of Year 1

such as grief, adaptation, choice and self-care. The organisation of Year 1 is shown in Figure 1.1.

It must be stressed that the processes (analysis, synthesis, clinical reasoning, decision-making, group functioning and maintenance, problem-solving) used by students when engaging with the learning material are essential to their learning, and at times these processes are not explicit in the documentation of students' work. As well, it is important to realise that a great deal of discussion, debate and questioning occurs throughout the whole process, especially when students share what they have discovered as they identify learning needs.

We will illustrate this process by means of a summary outline of what might be discussed in tutorial sessions and by commentary throughout the chapter, which will outline the structure of the students' week in relation to the *Timothy Randall* package. A framework is used early in the course to assist in each step of processing the data as a means of guiding enquiry. The development of this framework is described more fully in Chapter 9. The complete framework is shown in Appendix 1. The layout used in this chapter is designed to distinguish between different types of material:

- all work produced by students is in italics.
- material given to students to process is shaded.
- the processing framework, developed by facilitators and used as a guide, is bold boxed.

Timothy Randall – Block 1

Students have two weeks to complete the learning package *Timothy Randall*. The timetable for the package is shown in Figure 1.2.

Week 1

MONDAY	TUESDAY	WEDNESDAY	THURSDAY	FRIDAY
Problem-based Tutorial Block 1 (2 hours)	Biological Sciences Session (2 hours)	Problem-based Tutorial Block 2 (2 hours)	Infection Control (2 hours)	Review of Learning Package. Group Process (2 hours)
3 hours	1 hour	3 hours	1 hour	
Situation Review Tutorial (1 hour)	Behavioural Science (2 hours)	Situation Review Tutorial (1 hour)	Nursing Lab. Last Offices Infection Control	

Week 2

MONDAY	TUESDAY	WEDNESDAY	THURSDAY	FRIDAY
Problem-based Tutorial Block 3 (2 hours)	Panel-Support Group & Community Services (2 hours)	Problem-based Tutorial Block 3 Cont. (2 hours)	Nursing Laboratory Guided Imagery (2 hours)	Review of Learning Package. Group Process (2 hours)
3 hours	1 hour	3 hours	each group	
Situation Review Tutorial (1 hour)	Legal Issues (2 hours)	Situation Review Tutorial (1 hour)		

Figure 1.2: Timetable – Timothy Randall

This time-frame allows the facilitator and group some flexibility in processing material, although there are some limitations on this in terms of planned resource sessions for the total student group.

Timothy Randall is itself divided into three blocks. We will be giving you the opportunity to work on Block 2. In order to introduce you to this process we will first give examples of work produced by students in Block 1 of the package.

Finally, to give you a sense of the total package, the chapter will outline an excerpt from a transcript of an audio-tape used for Block 3 of the *Timothy Randall* package. The accompanying students' work follows as 'Notes to Block 3'.

Block 1

May 1989

Mr Timothy Randall, a high school teacher, aged 37, comes with his partner Colin to the Bougainvillea Ward at Yalta hospital where you work as a registered nurse.

Colin has been attending your unit for some months for routine tests to assess the progress of his Acquired Immunodeficiency Syndrome (AIDS).

Timothy and Colin have been partners for six years and have a close and loving relationship. Timothy has been waiting for the school term to end before they could move back to the city of Brisbane from the neighbouring city of the Gold Coast so that he can have his tests.

Both Timothy and Colin are very distressed on learning that Timothy's test is also positive for Human Immunodeficiency Virus (HIV).

Processing framework

A. Within the problem-based tutorial (two-hour tutorial)

Some crucial questions	Some useful prompts
1. Is there a situation in need of improvement?	• analyse the data • identify cues*

Issues

Timothy is a school teacher
Timothy is 37
Timothy has a male partner, Colin (for six years – it is a close and loving relationship)

Colin has AIDS
Timothy and Colin are very distressed → Timothy's test is HIV+
They are moving from the Gold Coast to Brisbane
Attending the unit for progress tests re Colin's AIDS
Attending unit for some months
May 1989

* The asterisked issues listed illustrate the cues, assisting in identifying situations in need of improvement, which students identified from the block material.

After discussing the issues identified from the block material the facilitator encourages the students to analyse them, determining why particular information is seen as important in examining the client situation. Timothy's being a school teacher may initially not be seen as an issue in consideration of whether there is a situation in need of improvement for Timothy. The students, however, gave reasons for seeing this as an issue, and the decision finally to accept issues is made by the group as a whole. The reasons students perceived 'Timothy's being a school teacher' as an issue are:

- this information gives some idea of Timothy's socio-economic status
- it provides some reference for Timothy's educational level
- there may be legal or ethical considerations involved.

2. What is/are the situation(s) in need of improvement (from the analysis of the data)	• write down this/these situation(s) • review this/these situations in need of improvement as they relate to the learning material

Situations in Need of Improvement

1. *Timothy and Colin are distressed about Timothy's HIV+*
2. *Colin has AIDS*
3. *Having tests in Brisbane rather than the Gold Coast, and wanting to move to Brisbane*

3. What are your possible explanations for these situations?	• list tentative hypotheses • which are the most likely hypotheses?

Situations in Need of Improvement

Tested Hypotheses
H = hold hypothesis
A = accept hypothesis
R = reject hypothesis

Students research the learning issues in class and in self-directed time, and after sharing this information the group discusses each hypothesis and decides whether it can be held, rejected or whether more information is needed to make a decision. You can see below how some of the original decisions were changed with further information: some went from being (H) to (A) or (R).

(1) *Timothy and Colin are distressed about Timothy's HIV+.*

It could be that:
*   *Colin feels guilty*   *(H) → (R)*
*   *Timothy might lose his job*   *(H) → (R)*
*   *They're afraid of dying*   *(A)*
*   *Normal reaction*   *(A)*
*   *They're concerned about how family will react (how to tell them)*   *(A)*
*   *Worried about losing each other*   *(A)*
*   *No cure*   *(A)*
*   *Financial stress*   *(H) → (A)*
*   *Transmission to others*   *(H) → (R)*
*   *Timothy will develop AIDS – not knowing when*   *(A)*
*   *Shock*   *(A)*

(2) *Colin has AIDS.*

It could be that:
*   *He will require specialised care*   *(A)*
*   *He accepts he's going to die*   *(H) → (A)*
*   *The disease is progressing rapidly*   *(H) → (A)*

(3) *Having tests in, and wanting to move to Brisbane from the Gold Coast.*

It could be that:
*   *Brisbane has better facilities*   *(H) → (A)*
*   *They wish to remain anonymous*   *(H) → (A)*
*   *They are originally from Brisbane*   *(H) → (A)*
*   *Brisbane was recommended to them*   *(H)*
*   *They were treated badly at the Gold Coast*   *(H) → (A)*
*   *They believe that they will be more accepted in Brisbane*   *(H) → (A)*
*   *They have family in Brisbane*   *(H) → (A)*

---

4. What do you need to know in order to confirm or reject these explanations?   • list learning needs

Learning Needs

    i   *HIV infection – progression*
    ii *AIDS*
    iii *Facilities available as resources and support*
    iv *Diagnostic tests*
    v *People's reactions*
    vi *Communicating with a grieving/dying person*

5. Where might you find what you need to know?	• identify possible resources • library videos, persons, experience, etc.

- *Library resources → journals, textbooks*
- *Blood bank*
- *Community resources, e.g. AIDS Council*

6. How will you best organise yourselves to discover what you need to know?	• determine resources to be pursued • plan your group's activities for self-directed study • decide how you will share this information with your group

Usually students, in groups of approximately twenty, process information from a block of learning material to this point in a two-hour session. The students are encouraged to determine appropriate resources for each of the learning issues before the two-hour tutorial finishes. The issue of resources is debated in terms of how appropriate they might be in providing recent, accurate, accessible and specific information to assist the students in testing the hypotheses generated for each of the situations in need of improvement. For example, students identified AIDS as a learning issue and the facilitator assisted them to work out what they needed to know about AIDS given this specific situation and the students' existing knowledge base. Students then were able more clearly to identify their learning needs – AIDS progression, tests, lifestyle changes and transmission. This in turn assists in determining appropriate resources.

Students also decided at this point how they would bring the information gained in the self-directed study time to share with the group.

B. Self-directed study (3–6 hours)
The group divided themselves into small groups (two to three people) to investigate the six areas identified in step 4 above. They divided themselves by nominating

an area of interest. On some occasions this has been done by pulling names out of a hat.

C. Situation-review tutorial (one hour)

Some crucial questions	Some useful prompts
I. How does the knowledge you have gained help you to confirm, hold or reject your hypotheses?	• share information • review hypotheses in the light of information

Some examples of the information displayed by students follow. These have been reproduced without change.

(I) Tests

1. *Screening – Eliza* – Enzyme Linked Immunosolvent Assay – Looking for antibodies in patient's (pts) serum. Add pts serum to antiserum to HIV, linked to an enzyme – Put on a plate with HIV virus attached to it. Antibody in pts serum will attach to antiserum on plate. HIV+ serum antibodies will bind to all sides. (Colour produced.) HIV+ no binding by serum – so enzyme linked antibody will bind. (No colour produced.) (2 hours)

2. *AGEN Simply Red Test* – unique conformatory test looking for glutination of red cells. Pts serum added to reaction serum and red blood cells. If antibody there – red cells clump together.

3. *Western Blot Test* – To detect which antibodies of virus are present – looking for 8 different antibodies – Fine strip of blotting paper with different parts of HIV virus on it. (1 week)

1 Further Test Eliza Method
P24 antigen test – looking for sera converters to P24 antigen – first antigen seen Beads – antibody coated and pts serum. If P24 antigen present will bind to bead. Colour reaction. (24 hours)
P24 antigen test also used in therapy.
P24 antigen first antigen to appear in HIV – disappears quickly – reappears in final stage of AIDS – therefore used by doctors to determine the final stage of AIDS.

Red Cross Lab – Eliza screens all donations – any positive referred to State Health Department.

(II) HIV

Stages: Uninfected, Infected, Development of antibodies to HIV, AIDS, dying, death

Three weeks to six months after infection with the virus, some people experience a mild fever which is believed to accompany the production of antibodies. T4 lymphocytes are destroyed by the HIV virus. T4 lymphocytes are mainly responsible for the body's defence against fungal, protozoal and viral infections and is also called cell-mediated immunity.

Major symptoms
– loss of 10 per cent of body weight in a short period
– chronic diarrhoea persisting for more than a month
– fever

Minor signs
– persistent cough for more than a month
– skin infections
– general itching
– recurrent herpes zoster (shingles)
– oral candidiasis (thrush)
– chronic herpes simplex
– swelling of lymph nodes

AIDS is diagnosed when a person has two of the major signs and one of the minor signs and there is no evidence of another disease affecting their immune system.

(III) AIDS

AIDS is a disease by definition. That is, AIDS is a combination of signs and symptoms. (A syndrome.) Some signs of AIDS are: a positive HIV antibody test, a diagnosed opportunistic disease, an alteration in the T4 lymphocyte count, enlarged lymph nodes, loss of weight and persistent diarrhoea. The symptoms of AIDS and of other HIV conditions include shortness of breath, fatigue, loss of memory and loss of appetite.

Full-blown AIDS

People who are specifically diagnosed as having AIDS are generally very sick, although at times they may feel well enough to carry on some everyday activities.

These people may be home bound and increasingly unable to care for themselves. They may have decreased or greatly curtailed their outside social activities and their gainful employment. In addition, they may be depressed or have symptoms of dementia or other symptoms of central nervous system involvement.

Persons with AIDS need evaluation and consistent help from a physician, pharmacist and dietitian. For many hours each day or possibly around the clock, they will need care from someone with knowledge or experience with AIDS prognosis and treatment.

Symptoms of AIDS

Loss of appetite	Swollen glands in neck, armpits or groin
Leg weakness or pain	Unexplained fever lasting more than a week
Night sweats (often profuse)	Painful blisters
Painless purple spots on skin	Dementia
White spots in mouth & throat	Loss of vision and hearing
Dry cough	Persistent unexplained diarrhoea

Students identify the sources of their information when they present it to their group. It is then possible to discuss the appropriateness of the text.

2. Do you have need for further information?	• list the questions that the group wants to have answered in fixed resource sessions

Questions

- *Some people have heard that there is a new strain of HIV that doesn't progress to AIDS?*
- *Function of the T4 cells*
- *Legal/ethical issues for a nurse caring for an AIDS patient, e.g., do I have to care for such a patient?*

In presenting the information gained about the identified learning issues in the one-hour situation-review tutorial, students are encouraged to ask questions and to link information with previous knowledge or learning. Two two-hour fixed-resource sessions are planned for the day following the processing of this block of material. For this package, the two resource sessions were (i) a biological sciences session where the first two questions were taken and (ii) a session on legal issues conducted by a nurse lawyer where the last question was answered.

D. Situation summary tutorial (two hours)

Some crucial questions	Some useful prompts
1. Will the knowledge you have gained enable you to accept, reject or hold hypotheses in order to make clinical judgements?	• review situations in need of improvement • review hypotheses

Please go back to the hypotheses listed for the three situations in need of improvement on page 16.

2. What clinical judgements can you make in light of confirmed, rejected or held hypotheses? (Clinical judgements are derived from the (A) and (H) hypotheses.)	• with further information, review situations in need of improvement • review hypotheses
3. What is the best way of acting on your clinical judgements?	Develop an action plan: • identify goals • identify ways to achieve goals • identify ways of reviewing your plan

As previously indicated, some of the hypotheses held were either accepted or rejected when reviewed in light of additional research/information.

Students worked in sub-groups to develop the action plans and presented their work to the rest of the group. The group and facilitator then discussed each aspect of the action plan to tease out such broad statements as 'reassuring the patient'. They were asked for example: What does this mean? How would you go about it? This can be done after students process each block of learning material or on Friday (see Figure 1.2) where action plans for all work processed during the week can be presented and reviewed.

The action plans for two of the situations in need of improvement are shown below:

SINI (1): Both are distressed

Clinical Judgement: They are distressed because Timothy has tested positive for HIV and they are now both facing death.

Patient's Goal:	*Timothy will have the best quality of life, e.g. better environment, best treatment available.*
Intervention:	*Timothy: To talk to him and answer any questions he might have; to find out about the treatment and stages of AIDS, and make him feel involved in Colin's treatment.*
	Colin: Treat him as a whole person and help him die with dignity.
Evaluation:	*Timothy will be more involved with Colin's care and be more informed about his condition.*

SINI (2): Colin has AIDS

Clinical Judgement:	*Colin has full-blown AIDS and Timothy has been diagnosed with HIV.*
Patient's Goal:	*Colin and Timothy will be as comfortable and happy as possible for the remainder of Colin's life.*
Nurse's Goal:	*To maintain a safe environment for himself/herself and Colin and Timothy, and to provide the support and care needed to both Colin and Timothy.*
Action Plan:	*To attend to Colin's physical and emotional needs; to encourage family interaction, and offer support to Timothy; to help maintain Colin's lifestyle for as long as possible.*

After considering the process and outcomes for Block 1, we would like to offer you opportunity of processing Block 2 of the *Timothy Randall* learning package using a similar framework to that used by students for Block 1. The student group's work is detailed in notes to Block 2.

Block 2

December 31, 1989: Bougainvillea Ward

Today you have been caring for Colin. He was unconscious for two days and died a short time ago. Colin's family, Timothy and some friends have been with him throughout this time.

You enter Colin's room and find Timothy inconsolable, repeating the words 'my life is over and I have nothing to live for'.

Timothy Randall – Block 2

We invite you to work through Block 2.

Processing framework

A. Problem-based tutorial

Some crucial questions	Some useful prompts
1. Is there a situation in need of improvement?	• analyse the data • identify cues
2. What is/are the situation(s) in need of improvement?	• write down this/these situation(s) • review this/these situations in need of improvement as they relate to the learning material
3. What are your possible explanations for these situations?	• list tentative hypotheses • which are the most likely hypotheses?
4. What do you need to know in order to confirm or reject these explanations?	• list learning needs
5. Where might you find what you need to know?	• identify possible resources • library videos, persons, experience, etc.
6. How will you best organise yourselves to discover what you need to know?	• determine resources to be pursued • plan your group's activities for self-directed study • decide how you will share this information with your group

B. Self-directed study (3–6 hours)

C. Situation review tutorial

Some crucial questions	Some useful prompts
I. How does the knowledge you have gained help you to confirm, hold or reject your hypotheses?	• share information • review hypotheses in the light of information

2. Do you have need for further information?	• list the questions that the group has answered in fixed resource sessions

D. Situation summary tutorial

Some crucial questions	Some useful prompts
I. Will the knowledge you have gained enable you to accept, reject or hold hypotheses in order to make clinical judgements?	• Review situations in need of improvement • review hypotheses

2. What clinical judgements can you make in light of confirmed, rejected or held hypotheses?	• with further information, review situations in need of improvement
3. What is the best way of acting on your clinical judgements?	Develop an action plan: • identify goals • identify ways to achieve goals • identify ways of reviewing your plan

Block 3 is presented as an excerpt from an audio-tape with Timothy. The work students produced from this block is detailed in notes to Block 3.

Timothy Randall – Block 3

Nurse: Could you tell me about the history of your being HIV positive?

Timothy: I was diagnosed positive at the end of 1988 and I had not considered that this would happen to me beforehand. My companion I was living with at the time – well the only companion I have ever lived with, he started to fall sick and started having night sweats, and so we thought – you know – that the unbelievable was going to happen. We went along and got ourselves tested at the medical unit in Brisbane – we were living at the Gold Coast at that time, he'd just moved down there... So he was tested positive and ... the next day, I went and was tested and the result came back positive and I really hadn't expected this because you know I was very career minded, and suddenly it was a consideration of what was going to happen to both of us – to our lives really – and the one thing is that we never ever apportioned blame to the other because we never thought that that was an issue ...

I remember that Christmas was extremely difficult for our families because my friend had to tell his parents and I had to tell mine, and I'd actually had a run in with them ... I just had to tell my parents that this was the score that I was HIV and that Colin had fallen sick. That was really a great shock to them. I remember it was tears on the phone. I'd always got on really well with my parents beforehand and it just doesn't bear thinking about. We never talk about it any more, because it was just too painful for my mother. She never ever makes arrangements about Christmas now – ever ...

Nurse: So what was that like for you?

Timothy: Well I found it incredibly difficult ... There was no way we could alter anything, that was the important thing, we couldn't change anything, so we simply had to make the best of what was there, and that is what drew my companion and I together, the fact that we were both very positive in attitude. That kept us going I suppose and it really kept us going all that year as well.

So we moved back to Brisbane because we couldn't rely on the Gold Coast to provide medical support. It had a terrible name and we refused to have anything to do with anyone down there.

Nurse: Was it that they didn't know anything about AIDS, or was it that you felt that you were discriminated against down there?

Timothy: Oh absolutely, they just couldn't cope with HIV or AIDS at all ... my friend had to go along to a doctor to get sickness benefits, and the doctor said 'Look mate just tell me what it is, what are all the symptoms, and I'll just sign it. I know nothing about this.' ... That was at the end of 1988 and we found that really worrying.... So back to Brisbane it was ...

Nurse: So in essence you were able to be together to the end?

Timothy: Yes, the great thing about that year was that we were actually together for a year day in and day out, and because I'd explained my situation to the superannuation they were actually paying me. I was on incapacity compensation they call it ...

Nurse: What sorts of things did the people that were caring for you both at the end do to help you deal with Colin's death?

Timothy: ... it was an incredible open-mindedness and there was no moral judgement made on our lifestyle at all. I think that was the greatest thing, that the nursing staff accepted us for what we were ... But there was no moral judgement, there was never any concern of how you got into this predicament. This was the stage that you were at and they were there to provide really supportive care and as a result that came through in their attitude, you know, in their actions, they did everything for us ...

Nurse: How did you cope immediately after Colin's death? What sorts of things made it easier for you?

Timothy: Very difficult time, I'd like to think that I was really sensible about it and I think I probably was, considering what had happened but I think the greatest thing was support that the nurses had given me, support that my family and friends had given me but I also saw a psychiatrist and we'd actually been seeing him because we'd had a few problems towards the end and so we decided that as a pair we should see someone for help ...

Nurse: What sorts of things do you do to keep you healthy?

Timothy: Now that I've gone back to work, I think I have to be particularly careful because before it was lots of sleep when I wanted to. Lots of support – I'm a very social person so I see lots of people and that is support enough for me. Now that I've gone back to work I get a massage once every two or three weeks and I know these things are expensive and that's a problem but I'm back at work so that I can actually afford them now, I have to get the priorities right. Luckily I went overseas at the beginning of the year, that was part of it. I wanted to see a few friends, just in case anything happened. I went to see a few friends so that was important ... Just in terms of relaxation because teaching is so stressful and I know that I have to take time out to say 'stop doing it, slow down, take stock, do something about it.' ...

Nurse: Could you talk about some of the tests that you have to have?

Timothy: ... But now really it's only my T4s that are really important because T4s are – it's basically my immune system which of course is the basis of HIV and AIDS – developing AIDS and if my T4 count is low then my body is susceptible to catching illness, catching diseases, so if my T4 count is high then that suggests that my immune system is in pretty good condition and that I am able to fight off flu's and whatever ...

Nurse: How difficult has it been to be gay in this community and what has it been like to have to pretend all the time?

Timothy: Yes sure. As I said to you before I think I've led a fairly charmed existence and because I had taught for about nine years by the time I actually resigned or left – and I think being gay and being a high-school teacher provides peculiar problems and I found that in the first year in whatever school I am in I have to sort of survive the name calling, and it's usually by a minority of people and invariably it's from kids – males particularly – whom I don't teach, so I seem to be a bit of a target for them when I arrive and because I tend to be fairly good at the job I build up enough respect in the school in that year to have that stop ... I know some people, a friend of mine who has actually lost his job because he was in a catholic school and was actually thrown out because he was seen at a gay bar in town by a couple of kids at school.

Nurse: Does that make you feel angry?

Timothy: No I don't because I think I was born in Queensland, brought up in Queensland ... they are the rules, they are simply the rules that you learn to exist by and I accept that. I do accept that. Being gay has never had anything to do with my teaching and that's always been important for me that I've always been incredibly professional and never the twain shall meet. I guess I just had to look after my private life and be very careful ...

Nurse: Could you talk a little bit about support groups and how important support is to you at this time?

Timothy: I think I am in a very good position because number one that I'm financially secure, which I think is so important because most people I know when you are struck down as it were, when you are, you are often young, or you haven't had time to establish yourself in terms of buying a house, so many people have been renting – they can't afford to pay for rent on their unemployment or sickness benefits or whatever they are on, an invalid pension for example they simply can't afford to pay it so it becomes difficult for them. So I think that Colin and I were really in a very good position, so that the support groups that I relied on were mainly family, particularly friends I think ... the District Nursing Service was just fabulous and I would have no hesitation in calling them up again when I fall sick ... All the services that Queensland Aids Council provides, cleaning your house, buddy system whatever, there's that, and also I've started going to Queensland Positive People (QPP), just on a purely social basis ...

Nurse: When you think about your own death what are your feelings, and how have you prepared for that event?

Timothy: Absolutely, I have got this all worked out, it's interesting because for me after Colin died I was absolutely totally prepared for death because, I guess because, he had gone and I wanted to go with him, and I really would have liked that ideal situation because I've had a good time and I'm absolutely prepared for everything that's going to happen . . . There is a folder in my cupboard and I say to my mother and father it's the blue folder and I've organised wills, I've organised my epitaph, I've organised everything so that it's all done. My psychiatrist says that if I fall sick then maybe it will be a different kettle of fish and that I'll look at death differently and I don't know that I will because I'll go quickly I think – I'd like to think that anyway . . .

Nurse: Given that AIDS is endemic do you think there are any political initiatives that should be taken by government?

Timothy: I think being involved with education I think that's the key to everything. Education is absolutely the key to everything . . . within the schools, and I think there is absolutely a huge hole there for discussion of HIV and AIDS because I think that many people know that AIDS exists . . . maybe students at the school . . . know people who walk around who live on a day-to-day basis and they are HIV and they are not infecting anyone and they're not sick and they're surviving . . . For me it has to start there otherwise it's just too late, when you've got people of 15 and 16 who are HIV – it's too late for the others – so education is absolutely everything. I guess I say that not only because I'm a teacher because it's the key, it has all the answers.

Nurse: Thanks very much Timothy.

Conclusion

We hope that we have given you a useful introduction to problem-based learning; and that, in working through this chapter, you have experienced some sense of the pleasure students have in taking charge of their own learning. The structured processing framework is very useful to students at the beginning of a problem-based course. Once they have mastered it they are able to begin to engage with more complex issues which ultimately lead to their being able to make sophisticated clinical judgements well before they graduate. If things have occurred to you as you have been working through this chapter we hope that you have made a note of them and that your queries will be answered in the chapters that follow.

Notes to Block 2

SINIs:

1 *Timothy's emotional state*
   It could be that:

• *normal reaction*	A
• *not prepared for Colin's death*	H
• *didn't accept he was dying*	H
• *realised he could die the same way*	A
• *feels alone*	A
• *he's in shock*	A

2 *Family and friends' loss*

• *unresolved issues re homosexuality (guilt)*	H → R
• *may need counselling*	A
• *they have accepted the eventuality of Colin's death*	H

3 *Nurse's reaction to Colin's death*

• *feels she/he doesn't know how to support Timothy, family and friends*	H
• *first death*	H
• *has seen many deaths lately*	H
• *used to it and knows how to cope with death*	H
• *guilty he/she hasn't provided support for Colin*	H

Learning issues

A *Procedures for nurses upon death of a person (AIDS)*
B *Counselling and support for nursing staff*
C *Physiology of death*
D *Implication for families who have had a member die of AIDS*
E *Communication with a dying person/family of a dead person*

Research

Some of the information that students brought back to the group in relation to the learning needs follows:

A. Procedures for nurses after the death of a patient

Last offices

The purpose is to reduce the family's distress when viewing the body, and to prevent distortions in the body's appearance during later viewing at the funeral home.

The goal is that the body will be clean and free of all equipment used for treatment within one hour following the pronouncement of death. The body will be transported with respect to the morgue or mortuary.

After the pronounced death by a doctor

1. Contact any person involved in organ procedures (except AIDS patients).
2. Remove hairclips.
3. Replace dentures.
4. Wash hands thoroughly and clean any soiled areas of the body.
5. Wrap the body in a shroud or cover with a clean cotton sheet.

Cultural beliefs

Muslims The nurse should straighten the body and remove drainage tubes only. The family washes the body and prepares it. Organ donations and cremation or post-mortems are forbidden.

Hindus The family see to the body.

Jewish It is acceptable for the nurse to tie up the jaw especially if there is likely to be a delay until the body is taken away. The nurse can remove drainage tubes.

B. Counselling and support for nursing staff

We have a need to grieve whenever we lose something or someone in whom we have invested. It is similar for nurses, who, as part of their daily work environment, are confronted with dying patients. Nurses are forced to confront loss, not only of patients and families past and present, but personal loss as well. Caring for dying patients over a period of time, such as several weeks, or watching patients go home and repeatedly return, involves a degree of emotional investment and a feeling of grief that requires resolution.

A social factor that has long affected the nurse's ability to grieve is the assumption that the role of the care giver is to be emotionally strong. Nurses attempt to remain controlled and detached, thwarting the acknowledgement or resolution of feelings, because they are told that the feelings of ambivalence or guilt towards the patient are inappropriate.

The nurse too can experience conflict between wanting to cure the dying patient and yet wanting the dying patient to be relieved of his suffering, if it is lingering death. Harper identified the process of adaptation, i.e., intellectualisation, which focuses on professional knowledge and facts that at times emphasise philosophical issues. The professional then experiences a sudden jolt that forces her out of her intellectual haven into a confrontation with the reality of the patient's impending death and a realisation of her own mortality. Grieving is triggered for oneself and at the same time by genuine pity for the patient.

C. Physiological death

Body changes

Rigor Mortis: the stiffening of the body that occurs 2 to 4 hours after death. The lack of ATP in the body causes the muscles to contract and, in turn, immobilise the joint. It leaves the body 96 hours after death.

Algor Mortis: is the gradual decrease of the body's temperature. Simultaneously the skin loses its elasticity and can be easily broken.

Livor Mortis: discoloration of the skin. The red blood cells break down, releasing haemoglobin into the surrounding tissue. Tissues after death become soft and eventually liquefied by bacterial fermentation.

Putrefaction: generally there is discoloration of the abdominal skin in 2–3 days and swelling of the tissues and the formation of blisters towards the end of the first week.

Adverse Spasm: system when death occurs in conditions of high emotional tension and results in a contraction of muscles which is probably mediated by the central nervous system. The most common manifestation is seen in the hands grasping some object.

D. Implications for families

Following the death of someone significant, those who are left behind almost inevitably suffer a deep sense of desolation. The patient's family may feel afraid and anxious. They find it hard to watch their loved one suffering and difficult to understand their fluctuating moods and unpredictable reactions. They may fear their own ability to cope with death, to control their emotions and face the future alone.

Parents of gay men often have a double problem: learning simultaneously that their son is gay and has AIDS. If they do not know about his homosexuality, they have no time to face this issue before facing the AIDS diagnosis. They may lose control and feel that they have been deprived of information. Parents may feel that they have to hide the fact that their son has AIDS.

Persons who learn that their spouse or sexual partner is infected with HIV find themselves in a similar situation, and must also worry about their own HIV status. They often feel that there is no one to whom they can turn.

Action plan for Block 2

SINI 1: Timothy's emotional state

Clinical Judgement	Timothy's emotional state of feeling alone and shocked is a normal reaction when accepting the death of a friend and partner.
Patient's Goals	Timothy will accept Colin's death and his own mortality.
Intervention	To be there for comfort and support if Timothy requires it.
Evaluation	Timothy has accepted Colin's death and has continued to live his life.

SINI 2: Family and friends' loss

Clinical Judgement	The family needs counselling for their grief.
Patient's Goal	Timothy will come to terms with Colin's death and the family will continue normal relationships.
Action Plan	Allow the family to express their feelings about Colin's death (or suggest).
	Get outside support (grief counsellors, social workers) for the family.
Evaluation	Do a follow-up session with the family to determine whether or not they have really come to terms with Colin's death . . .

Notes to Block 3

Block 3 – SINIS

1. Communication with family
2. Attitude of health professionals
3. Managing stress of work situation
4. Community education requirement – lifestyle conflict
5. Financial security
6. Maintenance of health

Block 3 – SINI 1: Communication with family

Hypotheses

• Family didn't know he was gay	H
• Family's denial	H
• Family doesn't want to talk about it – their type of coping mechanism	A
• Timothy feels closer to friends than family	A
• Doesn't want to get too close to family because he is dying and will hurt them by his loss	H
• Feels like he has already upset them enough – only just told them he's gay, now he's HIV as well	H
• Family doesn't know how to support him	H

Clinical judgement

Timothy's lack of communication with his family is due to his family not wanting to talk about HIV and he feels closer to his friends than to his family.

Action plan

Nurse's Goals   for Timothy to feel comfortable and accepted talking to his family

Client's Goals   as above

Interventions

- suggest group (family) therapy
- suggest each party to speak to medical authority (re nurses, doctors) separately
- suggest he bring this up with his psychiatrist

Evaluation   ask Timothy about communication with family and how implemented action plans were successful or unsuccessful.

Block 3 – SINI 2: Attitude of health-care professionals

Hypotheses

- Lack of education
- Homophobic nursing staff – morality or lifestyle reasons
- Staff refuse to work with AIDS patients for fear of coming into contact with contaminated substances

Clinical judgement

There is a definite need for AIDS education in modern nursing courses, and a possible need for nurses to undergo refresher training courses to upgrade their knowledge/skills on new issues such as AIDS.

Action plan

Nurse's goal   To be educated, competent and up-to-date in giving care to AIDS patients.

Block 3 – SINI 3: Stress management

Hypotheses
- To be able to cope with returning to work
- To maintain his positive attitude
- To be able to cope with his sickness/knowledge of death when the time comes.

Clinical judgement

Timothy should seek help in learning stress management skills so he can cope with his return to work and so he can maintain his positive attitude right up until his death. This will take some of the responsibility off his family/friends.

Action plan

Client's Goal   To deal with any crisis with a minimum of stress.

Nurse's Goal   To facilitate and educate him in his management of stresses, especially those involved with work.

Interventions

- He should identify all the stresses he thinks he will have to face – remembering Colin's death.
- Make use of support groups.

Block 3 – SINI 4: Community education requirement – lifestyle conflict

Hypotheses
- Because he is being discriminated against in the workforce and health care
- Because he sees the lack of knowledge about HIV/AIDS of the students at school
- To stop the spread of the disease.

Clinical judgement

Timothy feels discriminated against because of community attitudes and his own feelings.

Action plan

Nurse's Goal	To practise patient and community education in all settings.
Patient's Goal	To feel less discriminated against and less anxious.
Interventions	Actively not discriminating, educating patients, behaving non-judgementally.
Evaluation	Timothy feels less uncomfortable integrating his sexuality into his whole life.

Block 3 – SINI 5: Financial security

Timothy worries that there is lack of financial security for AIDS/HIV sufferers.

Hypotheses

- Worried about quality of life for those not financially secure.   A
- Timothy understands financial requirements from experience.   A
- Timothy feels that there is not enough government financial support.   A
- Because of their age, Timothy feels young AIDS sufferers haven't
  had the opportunity to support themselves.   A

Clinical judgement

Timothy feels there is a lack of government financial support, especially for young people who haven't had an opportunity to make themselves financially secure, for AIDS/HIV sufferers.

Action plan

1. Highlight this problem to various support groups, i.e. Queensland AIDS Council (QAC), Queensland Positive People (QPP), People living with AIDS (PLWA), Community and Social Services (CASS).
2. Enlist their support in approaching appropriate government bodies.
3. Push promotion of AIDS/HIV education in younger age groups.

Evaluation	Timothy feels he has made a difference.

Block 3 – SINI 6: Maintenance of health

Hypotheses
• Ward off any infection	A
• Prolong life	A
• Better quality of life	A
• Feel better	A
• Lead a normal life	A
• Less reliant on support service and resources – not using them up	H
• Keep on working – maintain normal existence	H

Clinical judgement
Timothy has to maintain his health to ward off any infection to prolong life and increase his quality of life.

Action plan

Patient's Goals

• maintain a healthy lifestyle and enjoy his life
• to remain and lead a 'normal' lifestyle

Nurse's Goal

• educate Timothy in methods of maintaining a healthy lifestyle

Interventions

• encourage him to have regular check-ups
• educate Timothy on assessing his own health

Evaluation   Timothy understands the reasons for maintaining a positive attitude, healthy lifestyle and uses available support services.

Chapter 2
Developing a learning package

Christine Alavi

Learning packages gave an overall, total picture of the experiences of people in hospital or wherever. You didn't think of a client as being a single entity; where you think holistically about the situation and what you do to improve it.

Liz, student

Developing a learning package is a co-operative and enjoyable task. It provides an opportunity to develop the curriculum with input from everyone involved: the teaching team, who must ensure that the package fits the focus of the module and year in which it will be placed; those nurses working in the clinical area who will provide the clinical material that is the basis of the package, and who will review it once it has been written; and the teaching teams from previous and subsequent years to ensure continuity.

The curriculum was designed so that the first-year learning materials would reflect Health in Semester 1, Life Change in Semester 2, Health Breakdown in Year 2, and Complex Health Breakdown in Year 3. This configuration is shown diagrammatically in Figure 2.1:

What then to include? How could we be sure that we had dealt with all the common issues and problems which confront nurses in the clinical area, whether that clinical area is within hospitals or in the community? This chapter will detail the construction of a learning package from the gathering of material, the

	Semester 1	Semester 2
YEAR 1	Nursing and Health	Nursing and Life Change
YEAR 2	Nursing and Health Breakdown	
YEAR 3	Nursing and Complex Health Breakdown	

Figure 2.1: Organisation of three years

development of the learning package and its accompanying assessment items, the gathering of resources, the planning of resource sessions, to the production of a concept matrix, which maps the introduction and reiteration of concepts across the course, and the evaluation of the package. An example of a concept matrix is shown in Appendix 2.

Deciding on the learning package

Once the focus of the semester has been decided, the learning packages for that semester can be developed. In deciding what learning packages are appropriate a number of issues need to be considered. Since the course is both integrated (that is, knowledges which are usually presented as discrete subjects are integrated within the learning package as they relate to that package) and reiterative (that is, concepts are presented and re-presented throughout the programme, becoming increasingly more complex), it is essential to know what has gone before so that the knowledge students have already gained can be revisited and built upon.

For example, in the third year the focus is on Complex Health Breakdown. In previous years the emphasis on health, life change and health breakdown has given students the opportunity to explore many of the concepts to which they will be reintroduced in this year at a more complex level.

> *Learning packages give an overall, total picture of the experiences of people in hospital or wherever. You didn't think of a client being a single entity, you thought about the situation and what you could do to improve it.*
> *Sandy Fox, Year 2 student*

To find out what type of learning packages might be valuable in the third year we look back across the preceding two years' concept matrices to see if there are any obvious gaps. The concept matrix shown in Figure 2.2 gives an example of how the exposure to such concepts is mapped across the course. This particular example is taken from a learning package in Year 1 which introduces the students to Aboriginal health.

In planning students' learning for year 3, we saw that there was a need to expose them to situations where they could give nursing care to a range of clients, have an opportunity to practise a range of skills which they had been developing and do this while managing their time effectively and prioritising the care they would give to clients. It was decided, therefore, that the most appropriate setting from which to gain learning material would be an emergency department, where the issues would range from simple to complex, and where individual clients, as well as groups of clients, would need care.

Health/ health break- down	Human structure & function	Behavioural studies	Nursing intervention		Society and its institutions
			Theory	Practice principles skills	
K N O W L E D G E	The eye The ear	'Normal' behaviour – role expectation	Health Aboriginal health Prof. roles – transcultural nursing	Health assessment	Political & economic issues of health care delivery – government policies
S K I L L S	Examination of the eye and ear		Communication – culture- specific	Communication with Aboriginal people	Reading epidemio- logical studies
A T T I T U D E S		Values clarification Power Control Stereotyping	Values of health care team		Social values Norms Control

Figure 2.2:   Concept matrix for Aboriginal health package (2 weeks)
Source: Adapted from School of Nursing, University of Western Sydney, 1990.

A group was assembled from the nursing faculty together with biological and behavioural scientists who were also involved in determining how we would proceed. We agreed we would develop a single package which would span the semester, and which would incorporate the care of all patients treated within an emergency department over one shift. One member of the team visited the emergency department of a busy local hospital to speak to the charge nurse, and to explain what we wanted to do.

The register of patients visiting the department on each shift was made available and a day was chosen from it which included patients with a wide range of situations in need of improvement. The charge nurse confirmed that this would be a 'fairly typical Saturday afternoon shift'.

Guidelines for learning package focus

1 Is the primary focus on nursing intervention?	2 Is there opportunity to reiterate generic nursing practice?	3 Is there a mix of primary secondary tertiary settings?	4 Is the package representative of lifespan?	5 Is the level of sociology individual → global?	6 Does it take account of epidemiology?	7 Presentation acute/terminal nursing interventions
Yes – student situated in a clinic for Aboriginal people	Rural community Cross-cultural nursing	Primary	Adults and children	Individual Family Community	Yes Aboriginal health statistics	Prevention Health/ health breakdown

Such a process typifies the way in which material for a learning package might be chosen. What precedes it is an agreement with the clinical agency that such materials can be used provided that confidentiality is assured.

Constructing the learning package

The fact that real cases are used in packages which apply to the reality of clients with real problems is great. A problem-solving approach facilitates our clinical decision-making.

Jo, Year 3 student

Learning packages can be constructed using written materials, audio-taped or video-taped materials and photographs. A variety seems to work best so that students do not become bored with only one medium. Various media can also provide different perspectives on the situation, since in the real setting information comes from written, spoken and visual material. In all of these cases the aim is the same: to produce material taken from the real situation and containing triggers so that students in the role of the registered nurse are prompted to take some action.

One of the most useful pieces of advice that we were given when we were establishing our course was to be sure not to introduce any artefacts into the material gained from the clinical area. Although it can sometimes be tempting to invent some of the information so that students will deal with some aspect which the teaching team feel to be important, this is almost always unsuccessful because there is no supporting documentation in the patient's notes, and students inevitably realise that the information is fabricated. From the beginning of their work with learning packages students are placed in the role of the registered nurse. This is done deliberately so that students think of themselves in that role, and take responsibility for the decisions they make in it. In the package discussed above, for example, Block 1 begins with the sentence:

> *You are the registered nurse in charge of the Emergency Department at Southside Hospital.*

The learning material is written to give the students blocks of information with which they must decide how to deal. The material is designed so that it will allow the students to make decisions very similar to those they will need to make as registered nurses and allow them to transfer their processing to the clinical area. As part of this learning package the students will spend time in an emergency department, so the knowledge they gain in the clinical area will help them in working through the learning package, and vice versa. Block 1 of the package described thus far reads like this:

You are the Registered Nurse in charge of the Emergency Department at Southside Hospital on the morning shift (7.00 am–3.30 pm) on Friday, 15th January 1993. Working with you this morning are:–

Tom Rimmer	a Registered Nurse who has worked in A & E for 4 months.
Jenny Todd	a Registered Nurse who has worked in A & E for 2 weeks.
Cassie Reynolds	a Registered Nurse who has worked in A & E for 7 months.
Margaret Pritchett	a Registered Nurse who has worked in A & E for 5 years as the Triage Nurse.

Maria Castro	an enrolled Nurse who has worked in A & E for 4 years.
Dana Pedero	an enrolled Nurse who has worked in A & E for 8 months.
Lyn Holmes	a Registered Nurse who has worked in A & E for 8 months.
Terri McAndrew	a Registered Nurse who has worked in A & E for 2 months.
David Cooper	a Registered Nurse undertaking a Critical Care Course.

Sue Attaway,)	
Tony Appleyard,)	
Ben Humphries,)	3rd year university nursing students
Samantha Clifford)	

Tim Reynolds was admitted at 5.00 am with a sub-dural haemorrhage and is in Cubicle 6 waiting to go to theatre.

Harry Chamberlain is in Resuscitation cubicle number 1, and awaiting admission to the CCU.

David Hodge who was admitted with a head injury from a MVA is presently at X-Ray and will return to cubicle 7.

You allocate the nurses to areas within the department bearing in mind that:

Room 4 is used for a fracture clinic until 12.30 pm this afternoon; and that Room 3 is used as a hand clinic from 9.00 am and as a dressing clinic from 8.00 am–11.30 am.

You do not, however, need to provide staff for these clinics.

As Damien, a Year 3 student, says:

> *This style of thinking and processing certainly makes one approach clinical with the feeling that it's quite OK not to know everything – nobody does – and if you don't know you can always find out. Looking at clients with an open mind and a non-judgemental attitude with an aim of restoring/maintaining health has become developed from PBL, and I intend to carry that through my professional practice.*

Along with this block, students were given a floor-plan of the emergency department, and a list of thirty patients and the times at which they had come to the department.

The original admission sheets and clinical file material, including assessment sheets, observation sheets, pathology reports and X-ray reports, were also provided to students so that they had full information on which to base their nursing care. Similar resource materials accompany other learning packages to amplify the information and provide further learning triggers.

In order to make sure that as wide a range of situations as possible is presented to the students, the concept matrix outlines the inputs into the package from biological science; behavioural science; ethics; legal issues; nursing; and the humanities. Learning packages should reflect an appropriate mix of primary, secondary and tertiary interventions, and should represent the lifespan from birth to death; there should also be an appropriate mix of gendered material in the course, and learning materials must take account of different cultural and ethnic groups. Refer to the guidelines in Figure 2.2.

Format of the learning package

The learning package is the main prompt for student learning. As such it is the guide to how students will structure their learning, and will indicate the resources available to help them.

The first page of the package indicates to students how they might organise their time. It outlines the times and number of fixed resource sessions, and the number of blocks of learning material in the learning package, as well as the clinical experience which will enhance it. A typical introductory page for a learning package, this time from a learning package in Year 2 where students are examining, for example, concepts of health breakdown in children, parental responses, conflict and nursing responses, might look like this:

Introduction

This package has been designed to enable you to examine concepts and issues related to Bruce Wayne's situation.

Organisation

Your exploration of this package will centre on the tutorials complemented by self-directed study and fixed-resource sessions.

Labs

Labs will be structured to enable you to focus on issues related to Bruce Wayne and his family's situation. Labs will take place on the Monday of week 2 & 3.

Components

Block 1, 2 and 3.

Figure 2.3:   Introductory page for a learning package

The next page reiterates the core concepts for the module, and provides space for students to record the concepts which they explore in working through the learning package. Figure 2.4 shows such a page.

Block 1 of the learning package is then presented. It may take the form of written material in Bruce Wayne, Block 1, or it may direct the students to listen to an audio- or video-tape. Generally, resource notes will accompany each of the blocks of trigger material. In this block the students have access to the referral letter from the boy's general practitioner, as well as the initial assessment on admission. Such resources are not distributed as a matter of course, but only when

Concepts and Issues

Core Concepts
- ▶ Change
- ▶ Adaptation
- ▶ Self-care
- ▶ Health maintenance
- ▶ Control
- ▶ Ethics
- ▶ Quality of life
- ▶ Coping
- ▶ Equilibrium/disequilibrium
- ▶ Enablement
- ▶ Stigma

On completion of each block use the space below to record the concepts you have explored.

Block I	Block 2	Block 3

Figure 2.4:   Core concept page

students can indicate that they need them in order to test the hypotheses they make about situations in need of improvement.

Subsequent blocks are presented in the same way, with accompanying resource notes, test results, nursing notes and so on.

These block materials were derived from discussion with a registered nurse, the child's mother and the child. The child chose the name 'Bruce Wayne' (Batman) as his alias for this learning package. A further Block 4 might be added after the child went on to have a renal transplant.

Bruce Wayne – Block 1

23.12.90 0650 hrs

You meet an ambulance as it arrives in the ambulance bay attached to the A and E unit where you work. As the ambulance officers open the rear doors you see a boy, who looks 5 or 6 years old lying quietly on the stretcher with his eyes closed and a distressed, crying woman is sitting by his side.

The ambulance officer tells you that this is Bruce Wayne, aged 8 years, who had two seizures at home this morning, the last at 0630hrs which 'was prolonged'. His mother, Donna has accompanied him.

You direct everyone into the trauma room and help transfer Bruce to the trolley bed. He is making incomprehensible sounds and pushes your hand away aggressively when you try to turn him onto his side. He starts to cough and then vomits onto the bed. His mother continues to weep.

Bruce Wayne – Block 2

23.12.90 2230hrs. Paediatric Intensive Therapy Unit, Nathan Hospital

Following the handover you are assigned by the Clinical Nurse Consultant (CNC) to care for Bruce Wayne who had a Tenckhoff catheter inserted last night. When you go to see him you find that he is crying. 'I want Mum,' he says to you when you ask him what's wrong. You sit on the edge of the bed and try to comfort him. As you are sitting you look around at the equipment that surrounds his bed. You are familiar with most of it but you are becoming increasingly agitated about the peritoneal dialysis (PD). You read about it a long time ago but you seem to remember nothing. The unit is running at minimum staff levels because it's Christmas and you don't know if the CNC will get back to you before you have to do anything with the dialysis.

2300hrs

Although now less upset, Bruce is squirming in the bed and complaining of severe discomfort all over his 'tummy'. You notice that his abdomen is distended and when you check his PD drainage tube there is no fluid moving in it.

24.12.90 0600hrs

Mrs Wayne arrives to see Bruce. She tells you that she's sorry she's come so early but she couldn't wait any longer. When she sees his peritoneal dialysis is connected and running she appears shocked. 'Have they started the dialysis already? I thought he was going to be transferred to the Dialysis Unit to start this. Isn't that the specialist place for it? No-one told me he would be having it here.'

Bruce Wayne – Block 3

13.06.92 1600hrs

You are a registered nurse who has recently transferred to the intermediate ward at Nathan Children's Hospital. You have been allocated to Bruce Wayne who is arriving at 4.15pm for peritoneal dialysis. Bruce arrives accompanied by his mother and two younger brothers. You notice that Bruce is approximately 20 cm shorter than his younger brother who is 9 years of age. You introduce yourself to Bruce and his family and sense some apprehension on Mrs Wayne's part. She makes minimal eye contact whilst you are speaking and only gives minimal verbal responses. Bruce is very quiet.

1645hrs

Bruce has commenced peritoneal dialysis and is sitting on his bed playing with his two brothers. There is some commotion from their direction and you walk over only to discover that Bruce's peritoneal dialysis has become disconnected with dialysis fluid flowing freely into Bruce's bed. You attempt to clamp off the bag. Mrs Wayne comes alongside you, realises what is happening and clamps off the Tenkoff catheter from which fluid is also leaking. She states angrily: 'Perhaps you should go and get someone else.'

1730hrs

Bruce has been reviewed by the medical officer who has ordered Gentamycin be added to the dialysis fluid. The dialysis is now flowing normally. You sit down beside Bruce and try to talk to him. He is very quiet and answers you softly. You notice that his dinner is sitting untouched on his bed tray. When ask about it he says: 'I don't want this.'

Mrs Wayne joins you after a while and states:

'I'm sorry for getting angry with you. It's just that I really worry about Bruce. If he gets peritonitis . . . well they can treat it . . . but it means he'd be taken off the waiting list . . . and who knows how long it would take before he gets a kidney. We've already been waiting for eighteen months. It's just that sometimes nursing staff don't seem to realise how easily he could get it . . . not that he's ever had it . . . I'm keeping my fingers crossed . . . but it would only take once.'

The teaching team involved in the development of a learning package will be a group of people who have expertise in the content area of the package, although they will consult systematically with others in related areas. For the Year 2 package described, the team comprised two paediatric nurses, a behavioural scientist and a biological scientist. Because other members of the teaching team may not have expertise in this particular area of nursing practice, the package development team produces a *Facilitator Guide*.

Concepts	Possible SINI	Possible learning issues
Equilibrium/disequilibrium	Boy on stretcher with eyes closed	How do you get to be on a stretcher
Human growth and development	Boy who is 5 or 6 is actually 8	Possible reasons for short stature
Coping mechanisms	Woman accompanying child is distressed	Crisis
Communication		Type of seizure
Stress response	History of seizures – could he have more?	Immediate neurological assessment → later investigations
Multi-system dysfunction in health breakdown	Full history not available	
Safety		Glasgow coma scale
Documentation	Boy makes incomprehensible sounds when disturbed	Obtaining case notes from previous admission
Homeostasis	Boy pushes your hand away aggressively	Identifying levels of consciousness
	Boy suddenly vomits everywhere	Anatomy and physiology of central nervous system
	Mother upset and demanding action	Signs of increased intracranial pressure
	This may be the time of shift change	Stress response
	Prioritising care	Care of the patient with altered neurological function
		Issues relating to verbal and written hand-over

Figure 2.5:   LP 1 – Bruce Wayne Facilitator Guide Block 1

Facilitator guide

The facilitator guide can take many forms. It may be a series of questions which might prompt student thinking; suggestions for the situations in need of improvement which students might identify; or a very detailed account of what concepts are built into the learning package, possible SINIs and learning issues. The format depends on the teaching team's needs as these are identified in discussion. The facilitator guide developed for Block 1 is shown in Figure 2.5.

Fixed-resource sessions

When the package is being developed it is possible to predict some of the fixed-resource sessions that students will need. For the Bruce Wayne package the teaching team identified that the students might need information on different types of seizures and their treatment; peritoneal dialysis, renal transplantation and the ethics of transplantation. Such sessions were organised, and experts were approached. The biological scientist and the nurse would give sessions on peritoneal dialysis and on different types of seizure and their treatment; ethics would be addressed by a humanities teacher, and transplantation by members of the transplant team at the local hospital.

In addition to these sessions, time is left aside in the timetable for students to have resource sessions on topics which have not been identified by the planning team. These are arranged on an *ad hoc* basis.

Nursing laboratories

Nursing laboratories are planned so that students can practise new aspects of nursing care, or refresh their minds about nursing care already encountered. Another chapter deals with this learning environment in detail, and it suffices to say here that the laboratories may have any focus which relates to the learning package in which they are situated. Laboratories are a safe place for students to practise psychomotor and communication skills before they deal with clients in the clinical setting.

For the *Bruce Wayne Package* described above the nursing laboratories could address neurological assessment, which the students have encountered in a previous package; peritoneal dialysis, which would be something they had not encountered before; communication with a child in pain and a distressed parent; and the nurse's responses to all of these situations. Laboratories do not focus on skills alone, but rather place the student in a situation in which holistic care must be considered as well as the nurse's own response. Students work in groups and thus have support from each other. The facilitator is on hand to help and support.

Other resources

Other resources which need to be planned and made available for the students to use as they work through the learning package are books, journal articles, video-tapes, films, games and computer packages. These can be made available in the library or within the school or department.

Evaluation

The learning package can be evaluated from a number of perspectives to see if it is achieving what the planning team intended. Once it is written it can be discussed by the whole teaching team, and can be returned to the clinical nurses who provided the original clinical material. Any changes can thus be incorporated before the package is used. This process is a very valuable one since it involves nurses with whom the students will be working in the clinical agencies, who can see that students are learning material which is relevant and up to date. Such nurses also feel some involvement in the development of the curriculum and are thus more likely to be accepting of students from the programme. As well, a review committee which has the responsibility for editorial matters will review the package to make editorial suggestions or changes.

After the students have worked through the package they can evaluate it and it can be re-evaluated by the teaching team. The student evaluation is important in discovering what the students found helpful or unhelpful, and what changes they would like. But it is even more important in convincing the students that they have a degree of control over their learning, and that the teaching team are concerned to take their comments on the learning material into account. An evaluation form which we have used is shown in Appendix 8.

It is also important that the teaching team spend time in evaluating the learning package as soon as possible after it has been used. Changes can then be noted and incorporated before the package is re-used. There has been discussion about how long the life of a learning package should be. We feel that after the package has been used for three consecutive years it should be replaced, because the curriculum as a whole needs regular review and because this is a reasonable time to check whether the package is still appropriate.

Learning packages can become a resource for other agencies. Some of the clinical areas which gave generously of their time and expertise in helping in the development of packages have used the material for staff development or in-service sessions.

Conclusion

Learning packages are the structure on which the processes of problem-based learning can be developed. Because packages are developed using clinical material they give the course credibility with the profession. They also provide for input from many members of the teaching team in order to produce material which students can work through safely before encountering it in their off-campus clinical experience.

Chapter 3
Facilitation

Gerry Katz

Having a facilitator was a wonderful experience. Somebody who would support you but encourage you to be responsible for your own learning. Who encouraged reflection and ultimately personal and professional growth; who recognised all group members and promoted a functional group.

Jody, student

Effective facilitation is essential to the success of an integrated problem-based nursing course which seeks to produce creative, independent thinkers and collaborative, self-directed practitioners. The profile of an effective facilitator has been likened to that of a saint: unfazed by ambiguity, undaunted by student irritation or personal frustration, whilst modestly eschewing credit for the learner's achievements.

This chapter outlines the path to sainthood by examining the nature of facilitation in problem-based nursing education and the multi-faceted roles and functions of the facilitator. Through the inclusion of evaluative comments from both students and facilitators, it is hoped that the reader will begin to see how and why facilitation is both challenging and rewarding. Facilitation and the facilitated learning experience refer to a method of teaching which transforms the role of the teacher and alters the teacher/student relationship. This discussion endeavours to highlight ideas and strategies for dealing with the transformation in the shift from a teacher-centred to a student-centred learning environment. It shares some of the common problems we have experienced in facilitating student learning, and some techniques for addressing those problems. The concepts and practical aspects of group process are emphasised and discussed at length, because these are at the heart of facilitated learning in a problem-based course. Little and Ryan advise that:

> The more skilled the tutor in facilitating group process and developing these skills in students, the less potential there is for group dynamics to inhibit learning. It is also more likely that students will use the group effectively and develop their own skills in communication and interpersonal interactions.

(Little and Ryan 1988:33)

In addition, some practical methods are set out to guide the facilitator who lacks expertise for the particular learning package being undertaken. All of these topics are offered not as prescriptions or panaceas, but rather as useful frames of reference for the reader.

Amending the teacher role

Much of the literature on problem-based learning points to the different nature of the teaching/learning situation. Little and Ryan (1988:33) state that, 'Perhaps one of the most significant implications of adopting problem-based learning is the need for change in traditional faculty/student role.' This observation is underscored by Wilkerson and Feletti (1992:3) who describe facilitation as a 'radical departure from the more traditional definition of teaching'. Barrows and Tamblyn (1988:11) noted that problem-based learning 'requires a different order of educational skills for the teacher who must be able to facilitate, guide and evaluate the student'. But, it must be emphasised at the outset, the concept of facilitation is not a denial of the notion of teaching. Margetson (1991:1) notes that 'teaching is sometimes contrasted with facilitation' and that, at the extreme, 'facilitation is opposed to teaching as when some facilitators deny that what they are doing is teaching'. Such denial demonstrates a lack of understanding of the role of facilitation in student learning. Facilitated learning is student-centred, and because it values process equally with content, and emphasises the development of self-direction and enquiry skills, one may (mistakenly) believe that the role of the facilitator/teacher is somehow reduced to that of a peripheral consultant who is, at best, marginally necessary. Nothing could be further from the truth, for as Margetson clearly states: 'The good facilitator is a good and educative teacher in so far as he or she facilitates valuable learning by students' (1991:8). This is reflected in the following student comment:

> *I have grown to prefer having a facilitator than a teacher, they provide help by questioning your decisions and really make you think. Facilitation allows you to be more responsible (compared to school where teachers spoon feed you).*
>
> *Sue, Year 3 student*

The nature of facilitation

The essence of facilitation (of any group or situation) is to create an environment in which the participants are free to define and advance their own learning goals, using their own creative energy to acquire whatever resources are deemed necessary.

Facilitation in a problem-based course means helping students to learn to trust their own decision-making and problem-solving skills and to give up accepting others' decisions about what is relevant or true. This happens in the various learning contexts, including the classroom tutorial, self-directed research, the nursing laboratory and the clinical placement experience. The facilitator is ultimately responsible for helping the student to integrate theory and practice, but the primary goal of facilitated learning is not the transmission of empirical data. Rather, it is to assist students to develop the requisite enquiry skills to identify what they need to know and how they may proceed to find it out. Thus, facilitation is a process role, one which is essentially the same whether the facilitator is involved with the group in examining the content of a learning package, in skills development, in clinical experience or in the evaluation of intra-group process. The role is one of assisting students to develop enquiry and decision-making skills, and fostering their ability to think critically in order to evaluate outcomes as self-directed adults. The facilitator *guides* the students through the enquiry and decision-making process, *questions* the rationale of their judgements and *challenges* their assumptions, and does so within the framework of an interactive group process. Ultimately, this leads to an understanding of the relevant issues, and skill in reasoning them, in a nursing context, to make sound judgements.

The learning package in process, for example, may be one in which the identified client is someone who has been diagnosed as having a schizophrenic disorder, based on apparent disordered thinking and seemingly incomprehensible verbalisation. Rather than telling the students the facts which (ostensibly) confirm the diagnosis, thus building the case for why this client is schizophrenic, the students are encouraged to question the certainty of such a diagnosis and to seek alternative 'truths' or possibilities through their own process of clinical reasoning. This process is equally appropriate to any clinical situation.

Such a process of guiding and facilitating both the processing of data and group process represents a dramatic shift in the locus of control in the classroom and in the clinical setting. As noted earlier in the discussion, it transforms the traditional teacher/student relationship, flattening the hierarchal structure and defining all those involved as participants in a process of discovery. Educators and nurses for whom the locus of control is important may experience discomfort in relinquishing that control, and some anxiety with the ambiguity and confusion which periodically surface in this type of learning environment.

As noted, many authors agree that facilitation is an uncommon skill among academic teachers; perhaps it is also a concept seldom considered by them when they think about what they do. Accordingly, the difficulties reported by many facilitators who express commitment to the methodology may be due to one or more possibilities. It could be that they are inexperienced; it could be that they lack a full understanding of what facilitation involves; and it could be that they have had no previous opportunity or encouragement to explore their value system as it applies to the teaching/learning situation. Thus, the transition from traditional teacher to facilitator requires the learning of new skills, making some important shifts in teaching behaviours, and a willingness to examine one's beliefs and values about issues such as authority, control, conformity, ambiguity, conflict, teacher–student relationships and the ego rewards in teaching.

We have all, to a greater or lesser extent, been imbued with ideas about the importance of an authoritative voice in the classroom lest chaos overtake; or that an egalitarian relationship between teacher and students sets a dangerous precedent; or that ambiguity, conflict and dissonance are anathema to learning. Letting go of these notions can be anxiety-provoking. Similarly, if our ego rewards derive from our role as the respected 'expert', we may be loath to give that up. However, interactive, egalitarian facilitation is difficult to practise if one's beliefs point to the opposite. But, as we know, it is possible to alter personal values and to change beliefs and behaviours; this is explored more fully in Chapter 7. The purpose here is to illuminate the value of facilitative approaches and the skills to employ them more comfortably.

It seems quite clear that effective facilitation mirrors the best of nursing practice, and that nurses who are able to reflect on how they may facilitate a client's return to optimum functioning or progression through to a dignified death need not be daunted by the practical aspects of facilitating student learning. Rather, they may find that, in many ways, facilitation of learning is a logical and exciting extension of what they do or have done in their own clinical practice.

> *Until you do it you don't have a real picture of it and when you do things fall into place . . . I felt able to capitalize on every learning situation.*
> *Jan, facilitator*

Co-operative learning and group process

As much as facilitation may be an uncommon skill among educators, effecting a co-operative learning environment is an equally uncommon skill among students. Most students have been educated and socialised into competitive systems which reward some at the expense of others. They have learned to work singularly, in their own interests, and to guard rather jealously their own research and production. It has been our experience, however, that as students become comfortable and adept with group process, they find the co-operative learning atmosphere fruitful, and in some cases truly exhilarating. This is borne out by comments such as:

> *In working with my group, people come up with outstanding pieces of information and questions the like of which I just don't know.*
>
> *Alistair, Year 3 student*

> *Working in groups can be at times very difficult and frustrating. However, it's real, it provides the skills needed to be a member of a health-care team.*
>
> *Tegan, Year 3 student*

> *In the beginning all I wanted to do was work on my own but now I much prefer to work in groups as it teaches you how to be assertive, how to be fair, participate, to listen. Working in groups is paramount in teaching you how to communicate and share the responsibility of learning. Problem solving in a group allows for more ideas and more options to be explored which enhances each student's knowledge-base and critical thinking.*
>
> *Kylie, Year 3 student*

Thus, one of the primary tasks of the facilitator is to create and foster a co-operative atmosphere in which collaborative effort is valued and understood. Such a task is made easier if the facilitator approaches it with a basic understanding of group process and group dynamics. Whilst it is not necessary to be a group therapist or an expert in the theories of group dynamics, an understanding of the different types of groups, their structure and processes, is certainly a requisite for effective facilitation. Such an understanding also contributes to the facilitator's ability to plan and design a curriculum and evaluate outcomes. With these factors in mind, the following discussion will focus on the process and functions of groups in problem-based learning, and the roles and responsibilities of the facilitator in the process situation.

Composition of the learning group

Ideally, the learning group should comprise no more than twelve to fifteen and no fewer than eight to ten students. A group of more than fifteen students is usually less successful because the more verbal or assertive members tend to dominate the discussion, whilst those who feel hesitant or unsure, for whatever reasons, find it easier to remain quiet and passive. Conversely, if the group is too small, the facilitator will find it more difficult to encourage enough diversity of viewpoints or ideas, despite the increased potential for interaction. This is not to say, however, that problem-based learning should not be implemented unless the ideal group size can be achieved.

One strategy for dealing with large groups is to subdivide the groups into smaller discussion groups within the tutorial, reconvening the large group periodically to share what has been accomplished, hypothesised or learned from the exercise. This may be done as often as the full group and the facilitator feel it is useful. The situation posed by an overly small group may be addressed by combining two groups and co-facilitating the tutorials. In our view, there is much to be said for co-facilitation; as with team-teaching and co-therapy, the learning environment is enriched by the added wealth of ideas and the example of differing viewpoints operating in concert. As well, there is the added responsiveness to student needs which two facilitators can provide. In any case, during the planning stages of a problem-based course, facilitators would do well to consider the optimum group size and argue for numbers as close to it as possible. Membership in the student group may be by choice or by assignment. In the early stages of a course, it is essentially random unless the facilitators decide to plan for a spread of age, gender, education, life experience and so on. Although students often express a desire to be in a group with their friends, experience has demonstrated that friends do not always work well or to each other's expectations in a collaborative learning environment.

Group process

The term 'group process' describes the actions, the interactions and the relationships of members within the group, which make the group a functioning whole. Group process includes defining or clarifying such factors as:

- the purpose of the group
- group leadership (who, when, how)
- expectations regarding members' contributions (including the facilitator)
- negotiation and setting of regulations such as how information will be shared, organising research responsibilities and self-directed time
- the need for 'time out periods' when the group gets stalled and how these will be instituted, and what will transpire
- the way the group examines and monitors its own process.

In problem-based learning, group process also includes the actual work of the group *vis-à-vis* the learning package: that is, the shared responsibilities and actions having to do with data analysis, collection of information, evaluation of the relevance and application of facts, further dissemination of information, all in a continual progression through to the end of the learning package. The facilitator *guides* the group in setting goals, in identifying learning issues and, if needs be, in organising the self-directed research so that it does not become unwieldy (especially important for inexperienced students). During the discussion of block material, the facilitator assists the group to remain focused and to reflect on the information at hand. The group may need guidance in framing questions for related fixed resource sessions; we have found that, if left on their own in this area, students often become overwhelmed by the task of selecting questions which will assist them to understand the nursing science concepts. In this activity the facilitator can help to demystify science (see Chapter 4).

It is essential that the facilitator *challenge* assumptions. Often the students are not aware that they are making assumptions when they speculate on such factors as how a client will respond or ascribe meaning to some behaviour described in the learning package. The facilitator advances the learning process by presenting alternative interpretations of what has been analysed and by relating the particular learning content to a wider social and political world. In their concern for factual accuracy, students often overlook or ignore the contextual relevance of information. The facilitator may be the one who reminds the group members to respect each other's input by listening carefully, and by critiquing it impartially and objectively. Students will learn that taking the time to do these things demonstrates the value of both the contribution and the contributor. One sign of successful facilitation of group processes is that this role will increasingly be taken by other members of the group. Brookfield describes group process succinctly when he states that: 'Learners and facilitators are involved in a continual process of activity, reflection upon activity, collaborative analysis of activity, new activity, further reflection and collaborative analysis, and so on.' (1990:10). And he notes that 'activity' includes cognitive and psychomotor experiences as well as the exploration of values and attitudes. (The reader will have encountered some review of this type of activity through the details of the learning package in Chapter 1, but we will refer to it again in one way or another throughout this chapter.)

The development of communication and interpersonal skills is also a significant learning task for students in a problem-based course, as these skills are at the heart of group process. Such skills include learning to give and receive positive and critical feedback, active listening, understanding and awareness of body language, the dynamics of verbal, non-verbal and incongruent communication, as well as gaining confidence in presenting or asserting one's point of view. The level of interpersonal skill among group members and the degree of sophistication in communicating will affect the group functioning. In general, we have found that the students' skills improve with time and experience, especially when the facilitator is a good role-model for these skills, and can provide a safe (non-punitive) and respectful learning environment in which to test them. The extent to which the facilitator is committed to helping students develop effective communication and interpersonal skills, indeed to developing these skills in themselves, will influence the success of the group. The effective facilitator is one who becomes skilled in posing questions which challenge the students to question their own preconceived notions or conclusions, as well as the reasoning process which drew them to those conclusions. (Examples of basic facilitator questions are contained throughout Chapter 1; others are offered later in this chapter.) Barrows and Tamblyn (1990:109) note that, 'At all times, the teacher must be aware of what he is trying to develop and shape in the student.'

Group leadership

This seems like a good place to say a few words about group leadership, which is certainly an important factor in group process and facilitation. The question of group leadership may seem to the novice facilitator quite ambiguous. Actually, it is simply that in some instances the facilitator is quite clearly the leader, while in others less definitively so and in others definitely not. The facilitator is centrally placed as the group leader in terms of deciding which learning package will be processed at any given time and how assignments and evaluation procedures will be designed and implemented, and in mediating the student's relationship with the institution. On the other hand, facilitation in problem-based learning lends itself to a democratic form of group leadership and one of the essential tasks of the facilitator is the encouragement of leadership on the part of the student members. While keeping in mind, and occasionally making explicit, the maxim that 'a good leader is also a good follower', the facilitator helps the group, by direct and indirect means. She guides the group in setting realistic goals, and developing strategies for achieving those goals, and by encouraging individual participation which is at once safe and challenging.

Little and Ryan (1988:33) observe that the facilitator helps the student to 'develop skills in critical thinking and problem-solving/reasoning, self-directed learning and self-evaluation . . . by questioning and challenging'. Clearly this represents a leadership role; those are skills which students will need in order to become effective clinical practitioners. They cannot be developed in isolation nor honed without the interactive group process. The facilitator is responsible for fostering and encouraging leadership behaviours among the students, to which some will be more amenable than others.

Whether involved in the evaluation of group process or in the activities of processing a discrete learning package, the facilitator must decide when and to what extent she will respond in either a *laissez-faire* or a directive manner. It is always an individual judgement which, with practice, becomes increasingly the one most appropriate to the group's needs at any given time. Confirmation of the appropriateness of facilitator behaviour in this regard will be found in the outcomes. The discussion progresses in a lively fashion with full participation of the group members, or the group process is completed with a general sense of wellbeing, or tensions which were present appear to have dissipated and organisational issues are readily addressed.

It is worth noting that, in a problem-based learning group, there is an admixture of formal and informal rules. For example, in working through a learning package, it is expected that the block material will be covered by examining specific material within a set timeframe. At the same time, it is also expected that each facilitator and group will bring their unique viewpoints to influence the way in which the material is approached and learning takes place. It will be important for the facilitator to help the group establish ground rules such as the participants not interrupting each other when material is being discussed and hypothesised. Some facilitators have attempted to set the rule that verbal participation is mandatory: a more fruitful expectation is that participation is mandatory and may take a variety of forms.

Brainstorming as a learning tool

Brainstorming is essential in processing the learning package, and it is this activity which many novice facilitators find unwieldy and difficult. To a beginning facilitator who is inexperienced in group process and who is therefore unsure of how to keep the student group on track, it may seem a fine line between being too controlling and not being directive enough. When one or two students seek to influence the direction of the discussion in ways that appear unproductive or wrong, the facilitator may feel helpless and frustrated. Facilitators, in their early stages of experience, have expressed concern and anxiety at what appear to be inordinate amounts of time spent 'flailing about in a sea of irrelevant ideas and opinions' expressed by students whom they see as having little or no acquired knowledge, either pure or applied. For the facilitator who feels that s/he has such knowledge, relevant to the situation under review, the impulse to intervene with 'correct' facts is superseded only by the frustration in believing it would be wrong to do so. When this is coupled with the expressed annoyance of some students who declare the need for facts and answers, the potential challenge and excitement of facilitated learning may pale into oblivion. But it need not be thus.

Encouraging students to become self-directed and convincing them and oneself of the validity and applicability of their knowledge and experience, however basic, is a bit like helping someone learn to tie their shoelaces. You may admonish them to watch while you do it for them, which is certainly expedient, or you may be involved by watching patiently as they work at mastering it, offering suggestions as they seem needed or wanted. It is easy to tell students what we believe they should know, but it is more effective, as students eventually attest, to facilitate learning so that what the individual comes to know is largely self-taught.

Brainstorming, in which ideas are welcomed uncritically in a set period of time, is an excellent method of stimulating group discussion. It is particularly useful for group members who are burdened with the expectation that all utterings must be correct and true. The group can decide what, if any, parameters – time limit, focus, etc. – will be placed on the brainstorming activity, and how the thoughts and ideas expressed will be recorded. It is a good lead-in to the process of hypothesising about the data in the learning package, and it is effective in setting a tone of acceptance and mutual respect among group members.

The facilitator has a vital role in assisting the group to take full advantage of the brainstorming process, by ensuring that the necessary subsequent activity of analysis, by sorting and critically reflecting on the material recorded during the 'brainstorm', occurs; but occurs without making judgements on the merit of the individual ideas. This is an important stage in the process; without it the ideas are wasted and students become disillusioned with the process, but unless it is carefully handled some students can feel reluctant to contribute freely in subsequent brainstorming sessions.

Evaluation of group process

An essential group function is the periodic evaluation of group process, a regularly scheduled time to look specifically at how the group is functioning as a group. This is done by the group members as they assess the actions, interactions, methods and outcomes which enhance or impede the learning process: in other words, what works and what doesn't work for this group at this point in time. We have found that a regularly scheduled time for this exercise underscores its importance and the need to attend to it. The approach can take any form and trying out a variety of approaches will help the students to see the advantages of different formats for different situations. For instance, the group may have an open discussion which is leaderless, or which is led by a group-appointed leader. From time to time, the facilitator may indicate a need to lead some or all of one session. Year 1 students and novice facilitators may feel the need for more structure, in which case the same format that is used to process a learning package may be employed to assess group process. (Is there a situation in need of improvement, what do group members hypothesise about the situation, what judgements, goals and plan of action may be made and undertaken?) Written feedback forms might be appropriate at some times, and other structured formats may be devised by the group, until such time as they become comfortable with a less structured approach.

Most people are able to distinguish between behaviours which promote group process and those which impede it, but it's not always easy, as the facilitator, to know how to respond in ways that won't inhibit further discussion, especially of the latter. One technique is to notice and make explicit what you see and hear going on in the group. Depending on what work the group is doing, it may be necessary to make a note to yourself and refer back to it during the process evaluation session. Or, it may be appropriate to call a 'time-out' and discuss the process. This is equally true whether it be a positive or a negative situation. An effective way to begin is for the facilitator to open the discussion with the words, 'I see . . .' or 'I hear . . .', 'I notice that . . .' and then the question, 'Does anyone else share my experience?' Such an approach invites students to agree or disagree, and to share their experience of what is occurring (or has occurred) in the group, without their input being designated either right or wrong. We have found that, as students see and experience the effectiveness of this kind of communication, they begin to integrate it into their clinical practice with clients and with professional staff.

Keep in mind that, in the facilitation of learning, it is just as important to observe explicitly when the group is working well as when there are problems: the facilitator can help the students to identify the reasons why the group's process is working well so that the behaviours can be reenacted in future sessions and eventually synthesised. Similarly, the facilitator will help the students to identify and rectify the difficulties which have impeded the learning process. Implicit in all of this is our belief in the importance of open, non-censorious communication and the facilitator as a role-model.

Process issues and the learning environment

As noted earlier in the chapter, we subscribe to the view that problem-based learning 'values process equally with content'. This viewpoint underscores the concept and practice of collaborative group learning which is so central to a problem-based model. In practical terms we have found that, if the (group) process is not working cohesively, then content cannot be effectively addressed and understood. In other words, people find it difficult, sometimes impossible, to learn or work when their interactions with others, and perhaps their sense of self, are impeded or impaired. One of our co-authors, Bob Ross, suggested the maxim: 'The process must be right for the content to be understood'.

As outlined briefly above, at such times the facilitator is responsible for helping the group to notice that group process is not working, and to define the need for some process evaluation. The process discussion may entail a brief aside to sort out a minor problem or disruption occurring in the processing of the learning package; or it may require a lengthy discussion about how and why this group is not functioning well, and what is to be done about it so that a co-operative learning environment can be re-established. The facilitator will need to judge how much of a leadership role to assume. As might be expected, the less experienced students require more guidance. As students gain confidence and sophistication, they become skilled at identifying the need to look at group process, and the appropriate point in time to do that.

The following are examples of situations in which the group process is interfering with the learning process, along with some suggested facilitator responses:

- the group is obviously uncomfortable with the content or focus of the learning package, but is not verbalising that discomfort. Issues such as sexuality, conflict and death are typically difficult ones for students to discuss. The facilitator is ultimately responsible for identifying and making explicit the group's hesitancy or difficulty, and helping them to work it through (to process it). This is an example of a situation in which the facilitator's own experience of similar feelings and how they were managed, can be related and used to good advantage. (Please see the section entitled 'Dealing with issues' in this chapter for additional strategies.)
- the views of two or three students dominate the discussion, and the rest of the group acquiesces, or sits in frustrated silence. The two or three may be potential leaders who need to learn effective leadership behaviours, or they may be students who are thoroughly unskilled at working within a group. Either way, the facilitator will need to draw out the views of the others. This may be done by reiterating the importance of hearing from everyone in the group, and the value of each person's thoughts and opinions. If such encouragement is not fruitful, it may be necessary to have the students break into smaller discussion groups and then report back to the larger group. The use of a hypothetical situation to explore the dynamics of this situation is also useful because it takes the discussion out of the realm of the personal. If the behaviour persists, it may be necessary to confront the process issues of why the group is deferring to a few members or letting them do the work of all. This will help the group to grow, through the experience of confronting and resolving difficult issues openly. The facilitator may also find it necessary to meet privately with the student(s) to help them with improving basic interpersonal skills.
- group members are consistently late, or attending the learning arena (tutorials, clinical, laboratory) sporadically, resulting in a continual review of what has already been covered, and thus impeding the group from moving ahead with their learning process. It is important for the facilitator, and ultimately the group, to understand that all behaviour is an attempt to communicate meaning, and that non-verbal communication is generally more significant than verbal. So-called 'misbehaviour' or opting-out behaviour is a signal that some members of the group are uncomfortable or unhappy. For the facilitator, it denotes

the need for process intervention. This may take the form of a 'time-out' to examine group process, and may begin with the general comment, 'I notice that people are coming late quite a lot and/or attendance is sporadic. I find this behaviour disruptive to the learning process. Do others in the group notice this, and what does this behaviour mean for the group?' The facilitator can help the group set limits on disruptive behaviours once the group has determined whether group process is at the root of it; that is: members are feeling excluded, devalued, having difficulty keeping up with the content and so on. It may be that personal problems require a private one-to-one discussion between a student and facilitator: this should always be an option, but not an alternative to the examination of group process.

- students feel irritated, annoyed, angry or dispirited with the problem-based framework and with the facilitator who continues to respond to fact-seeking questions with non-factual answers (e.g. Q: Why is the child in danger of developing pneumonia? A: What do you think about that?). If the facilitator has succeeded in creating a safe group environment, one in which issues and not people are judged on their merit, then some-times the simple venting of feelings and knowing that they have been heard is enough to allow the learning process to proceed. It is essential that the facilitator become skilled at guiding such discussions in ways that accept and value the input of each group member, and that she respond non-defensively to feedback which seems potentially negative. The facilitator who is skilled and comfortable in active listening will be able to lead the group process without needing to take charge of, or solve, the problems.

There are times when the cohesion of the group seems to be a figment of everyone's imagination, students refuse to participate in any discussion be it of content or process, some demand a lecture because the learning package is 'too complicated', group members fail to bring the results of self-directed study material to the discussion or simply don't do the research, some students seem incapable of synthesising any prior learning with what is currently being addressed, and on and on. Such situations happen in the life of every facilitator no matter what their skill or experience. It seems to occur once a term or semester, and, when it does, the temptation to revert to a standard, didactic form of instruction can feel almost overwhelming.

At times like these a facilitator support group and the freedom to call on a colleague for help are essential. Facilitators can support each other by sharing strategies that have worked in similar situations, helping to figure out what the group dynamic might be, and affirming that 'it happens to all of us at one time or another'. Facilitators may wish to help each other by direct intervention; sitting in to share observations about the intra-group process or acting as a substitute facilitator for one or two sessions with the regular facilitator remaining in or not, as seems appropriate. These are some techniques which can revitalise the group.

In such circumstances, it is really important to be reminded that all students, no matter what the course of learning model they find themselves in, experience periods of discouragement and feel simply fed up. Facilitator empathy about those feelings can be helpful. However, this apparent 'down-time' might be a signal that the group needs some space to put aside content and process issues, and do something different or unique for a session or two. This could entail several possibilities, with the group operating as one or in sub-groups which lend themselves to individual talents and interests. The students might be invited to make posters or a video, or devise a survey questionnaire to take into the community to interview citizens and government officials and report their findings to the wider student body. The possibilities are endless and limited only by the group's imagination: brainstorm it and watch the creativity emerge.

One of the excellent things about facilitating in a problem-based learning course is the tremendous opportunity for creative teaching and learning. Thus, what at first glance may seem like a dreadful low point in facilitation can, in fact, be a chance for the group to experience some new and exciting forms of co-operative learning.

The value of group process

Problem-based learning aims to teach students the value of co-operative decision-making and problem-solving, and to foster critical reflection about how knowledge is constructed and method is devised. These are not just interesting concepts but important to the practicalities of clinical nursing. Our experience tells us that students come at these ideas in varying stages of ability and readiness, and the nurturing that is required to help the students make them a reality can really be provided only through interactive group work.

Under the guidance of a facilitator who understands and demonstrates the importance of group process in problem-based learning, students become increasingly skilled at enquiry, critical reflection and interpersonal communication. They give themselves permission to say out loud, 'I don't know', 'Why is that?' or 'It could be that . . .' without fear of being wrong. We have found that, through the regular assessment of group process, students gain a clearer understanding of themselves, the motivation of others and the constraints – usually fear of ridicule or rejection – which can impede any one of us from speaking out or asserting ourselves. Participation in process analysis teaches that it is possible to exchange feedback and negotiate differences, factors essential to making informed decisions in the clinical area. We have found that students do take this learning into the clinical setting and discover that they can be active participants in the enquiry and decision-making processes for client care, instead of responding as the passive recipients of orders and directives. They are able to use the differing views they encounter to broaden their understanding of client care in the health-care setting. This is reflected in the following informal student feedback comment:

> *In my last clinical placement I was really able to see how what we do in these tutorials can be used out there. The nursing staff on the ward where I was working were arguing about what to do for this patient and people were getting pretty irritated. I told them about how we do group process when we are trying to figure out the patient's situation. They tried it and I felt really proud when one of them told me later how well it worked.*
>
> Isabella, Year 3 student

Dealing with issues

The facilitated learning process helps students to deal both cognitively and emotionally with issues in ways that are impossible in a lecture format or a question–answer session. Referring to the learning package set out in Chapter 1, let us examine how this can be done.

Some of the important issues raised by this learning package are values and beliefs about AIDS, homosexuality, terminal illness and death, and loss and grief. The facilitator might choose to open the discussion by asking group members to share their understanding and their views on HIV and AIDS. This call for participation might be initiated by facilitator-directed questions, but we would wish to emphasise the importance of the facilitator's reflections and stories of personal experiences in similar situations as a means of helping the student group to begin to discuss difficult issues. The facilitator will need to be aware of not dominating the discussion with personal tales, although, when briefly and cogently interspersed, these can be a useful role-modelling tool, as well as useful in generating group discussion.

- How have you experienced HIV and AIDS?
- Have you known someone who has been diagnosed, and if so what has been your response?
- Where does your information on HIV and AIDS come from? – friends? newspaper? person with the disease? relatives? medical resources? your family?
- How do you feel about nursing someone with AIDS? What are your concerns or fears? What are your responsibilities?

From the responses to these or like questions, the facilitator can guide the discussion to a consideration of the broader issues of sexuality and homosexuality with such questions and reflections as:

- What has been your experience of talking about sexuality in a group? How has that felt for you?
- How is the issue of sexuality a concern for nurses?
- What does society appear to think/feel about homosexuality?
- How do those views correspond to your own? How does the social value of an issue such as this affect the delivery of health care? How could you, as nurses, have an impact on this?

From this particular focus, the facilitator may select, or may see that the group is ready to move on to dealing with the issues of terminal illness, death, loss and grief. Such prompt questions as follow below will help to further this exploration of disquieting issues:

- How do you reconcile your nursing goals of healing and helping people to recover with caring for someone who is terminally ill?
- Are there specific or unusual issues for the client with AIDS?
- How does the nurse deal with the psychosocial issues?
- What has been your experience with loss? with death? with grief?
- How would you manage your own feelings in the face of the client's fears and concerns? the feelings of his partner and family?
- When and how do your feelings in the situation get attended to?

The facilitator might ask the students to keep some written reflection of their responses to these questions, and then return to them at the close of the learning package to consider how and why their views have or have not changed. The facilitator may wish to do the same, and to share his or her own reflections, knowledge gained, personal issues for future exploration, and so on.

As facilitators, we need always to be aware of the reticence that people may experience in dealing with such personal and emotionally laden topics. It has been my experience as a therapist and as a nurse that what is most personal is also most universal. Students seem reassured to learn this, and it is invaluable when they use it in their work with patients and clients.

How necessary is the facilitator's subject expertise?

Questions having to do with their own expertise are often posed by prospective facilitators. They want to know how their own expertise will be utilised in an integrated problem-based course and, conversely, how they will function when facilitating a learning package which is out of the range of their current knowledge or experience. The answer to the first query does in some ways answer the second.

It has been our experience that the richness of the learning environment in a problem-based course owes much to the integration of diverse backgrounds, knowledges and points of view. That integration occurs in a variety of ways. In the development of both the broad curriculum and the specific learning packages, faculty knowledge and experience are put to use to ascertain that the problem-situations will contain both relevant and realistic content. As we said in the Introduction, 'Problem-based learning is open to whatever considerations are relevant to dealing with a problematic situation' (p. 2). This accommodates a multi-focused learning package such as the one set out in Chapter 1. It is expected that the students, like professional nurses, will be dealing with myriad problems when faced with the holistic care of a client who is sick or injured. In this case – of a client diagnosed with AIDS and of the related issues for him, his partner and his family – a wide variety of nursing skills and knowledges will be required to process the learning package.

This leads to the second part of the question: how does one adequately facilitate student learning through unfamiliar material? For the conceptual part of the answer, the reader is once again referred to the Introduction which notes that problem-based learning 'reflects a significantly different conception of knowledge and understanding', one which eschews a conception of knowledge as eternally fixed. It embraces a 'more tentative character to knowledge, possibly an evolutionary character' as contrasted to something static and immutable. What this says to a facilitator is that a specific knowledge of all pertinent facts relevant to the content of a learning package is not required to facilitate student learning effectively. We have said that the goal of facilitation is to 'help students to think creatively, intelligently, critically and sensitively about the problem-situation in question [which] guides them where necessary and in a non-didactic way to knowledge' (see p. 3). Are we not then talking about a process of discovery in which both facilitator and student are active participants? In our experience, there are a variety of resources to expand and enhance the facilitator's knowledge-base. These include the resource material provided with the learning package, the expertise of colleagues and the material which students bring from their self-directed research of learning issues, as well as the expertise engendered through the fixed-resource sessions.

There are several ways to further the facilitator's process of discovery, to allay facilitator anxiety and to equalise, as much as possible, the students' learning experience irrespective of which facilitator they may be working with. These include a carefully constructed facilitator's written guide to the learning package (see Chapter 2) and teaching-team discussions which include a detailed review of the learning package before it is presented to the students. Ideally, this type of discussion will be the culmination of earlier planning sessions which involve the wider faculty. Intermittent discussions occur as needed among facilitators of the particular learning package, and an evaluation meeting is held when processing of the package has been completed.

A facilitator support group (see Chapter 7) is an excellent forum for facilitators to discuss both their problems and their successes in processing a learning package, facilitating the development of clinical skills and techniques for group process. It is acknowledged among colleagues that they can call on each other and/or refer students to each other in respect of expertise. The ways in which this consultative process is structured are entirely up to the team or the faculty at large.

Facilitation in the clinical area is addressed in Chapter 6, but it is worth noting here that a good deal of what has been covered in this chapter is similarly applicable to the clinical setting. Clinical facilitators frequently express some of the same questions and concerns about the nature of facilitation in a problem-based course, particularly as regards group process, self-directed learning and student self-evaluation. The elements of facilitation which have been discussed in this chapter are intended to assist or enlighten facilitators about the process, regardless of the learning situation.

The role of the facilitator in curriculum planning has been mentioned briefly, and is covered more succinctly in Chapter 2. It is important to be aware that the interactive processes in which we expect students to become proficient are a reflection of how facilitation skills would best be practised among faculty. In an integrated problem-based curriculum, the facilitator is at the centre of curriculum planning, effecting it in a collaborative, co-operative manner with colleagues, often with the same content and process issues which face the students. As facilitators gain confidence and skill, they are able to discern the parameters of an effective learning package. Problem-based learning is unlike some traditional academic structures in which a course is often devised by one individual and with limited opportunity to share its strengths and deficits with peers. As facilitators, we have enjoyed the collegial richness of shared ideas and perspectives, and the validation of our individual contributions.

Conclusion

In closing this chapter, it is difficult not to 'wax eloquent' about facilitation in a problem-based learning course, because my own experience of it has been so rewarding. Working within this learning model with both students and colleagues has confirmed my view that people do their best when they are given the opportunity to learn by enquiry and discovery, appropriating knowledge in ways that are relevant to themselves. Through the process of facilitated learning, students have the freedom and the responsibility to direct all the important areas of their learning. Personal autonomy is as much at the heart of facilitation as is co-operative endeavour. In the role of facilitator we become actively involved with the students on a journey of discovery, sharing equally in the responsibility for progress in learning. Along the way, we all discover things about the desired relationships between people: student and teacher, client and nurse.

I have watched students gain confidence as nurses, in tutorial groups, in laboratories and fixed resource sessions and, most importantly, in the clinical setting. I've watched them questioning and challenging, getting rebuffed yet refusing to be intimidated or silenced. And I have heard the admiration and respect accorded them by many professional nurses who, like me, were 'trained' decades ago.

Finally, facilitation is, in my view, simply the most logical and empowering way to teach – anything! This is best exemplified by a student who, on completion of the course, wished to express her appreciation to us for her facilitated learning experience. She proffered a small card in which she had inscribed the following message: *'And it was said of a great leader – we did it ourselves!'*

Chapter 4
Integrating knowledges:
the case of science

Michele Don

> *I have been able to place everything I've learned into practice. All situations are realistic and this makes the transition much easier – I feel that I have learnt the skills to identify a problem and know where to go to find the answers.*
>
> *Desaree, student*

While the presentation of the science components within any nursing course is intrinsically interesting, it can produce difficulties, particularly if it is dealt with by means of a discipline approach rather than through the perspective of relevance for nursing. In a fully integrated problem-based approach to nursing education the onus is very much on the whole teaching team to ensure that the underlying science principles are adequately addressed as students progress through the course. This chapter outlines the various aspects of integrating science within a problem-based nursing curriculum. Although the main emphasis will be on the biological and physical sciences, strategies discussed readily apply to facilitation of student involvement with knowledge within any integrated problem-based educational experience.

Integration at the design stage

At the outset the aim should be to demystify science, to attempt to explain concepts in understandable language rather than using technical jargon. In a fully integrated course it is necessary not only to overcome the division of scientific knowledge into discrete disciplines but also actively to encourage the overlapping of discipline areas. For example, the physics principles associated with pressure in fluids can be dealt with not in the rigid framework of the laws of matter, but contextualised within situations involving air movement during external respiration; pressure changes during intravenous therapy; blood pressure measurement associated with health assessment; or filtration in the glomerulus of the kidney, to cite just a few of the many instances of the application of these principles.

In a fully integrated, reiterative problem-based course, scientific knowledge is introduced as the need for it is identified, in major part by the students themselves. This should occur as they progress through discussion of learning needs associated with a particular learning package. These basic needs must also, of course, be anticipated by the faculty both in the design of the stimulus material and in the provision in the timetable for the necessary fixed resource sessions. Although, in the case of Griffith University Year 2, students themselves identified the need to know the basics when asked about 'how science fitted into problem-based learning'. However, they were clear that there was not a 'list of basics' as 'everyone . . . brings to the group different background knowledge'.

Package material provided to the students must contain triggers to initiate inquiry into scientific concepts underlying the situation under investigation. Such triggers may be clearly evident in the block material of a given package or they may be presented in accompanying resource notes which can be explored by the students when they find that they need such things as admission letters, pathology charts, X-ray reports, case notes, and so on.

The presentation of the trigger material within the blocks may take various forms depending on the particular package or time in the course at which it is presented. In some instances writing material may provide the most appropriate medium; in the following examples, the science triggers have been highlighted to illustrate the elements which are considered, in part at least, to comprise stimuli for science-related investigations:

- from a Year 1 package – both Timothy and Colin are very distressed on learning that Timothy's test is also *positive for Human Immunodeficiency Virus (HIV).*
- from a Year 2 package – you are also told that Mrs Sayer *spiked a temperature* overnight. She has been placed on *intravenous antibiotics for suspected pneumonia and oxygen therapy* was instigated. Other orders included: a request for physiotherapy and the administration of an *enema*. The enema has not yet been given.
- from a Year 3 package – on arrival at the emergency department he was *intubated but awake; his pulse was 60 and regular; his respiratory rate was 12 per minute and his B.P. was 100/70. His accompanying X-ray shows a vertical fracture through the C5 vertebral body.*

The complexity of this trigger information may appear from the examples above to increase as the course progresses. To some degree this may be the case, but triggers should, in fact, be presented in such a way that students are able to interpret and instigate appropriate investigations of them at whatever point in the three-year course they are introduced in a learning package. Prior knowledge will determine the degree to which trigger information requires further investigation outside tutorial discussions.

One of the principal aims of a course like this is that students will progressively gain the ability to identify for themselves the relevant learning issues. These issues should encompass all disciplines in order to facilitate an adequate understanding of the clinical situation in need of improvement and to enable students to formulate clinical judgements and action plans. Each student's prior knowledge helps to inform the group in making the identification of essential learning needs. Group interaction and sharing may alleviate some of the extra demands that certain educators believe an integrated curriculum places on students. As Grady (1984:323) states, 'An integrated curriculum demands more of students in that it often requires them independently to acquire facts specific to a given situation, and also presupposes their capacity to learn to differentiate, integrate and generalise from knowledge.'

To enable students to learn effectively in this way it is therefore essential that, in the preparatory stages of assembling a learning package, there should be wide consultation with people representing a cross-section of the discipline areas addressed within the package. This should ensure that information to stimulate relevant learning issues is included within the triggers of the package and that resource sessions with appropriate experts are included in the final timetable. The completed learning package should ideally be previewed by everyone who is to be involved in its implementation before it is presented to the students – see Chapter 2. Often this is not practical if an expert is being used only once, but this person should at least have access to whatever material the students are processing before presenting their resource session.

Practising integration

There are distinct advantages if the science sessions within an integrated problem-based learning course can be presented, in most part, by a limited number of specialist staff dedicated to an eclectic approach to the science education of nurses. This approach allows for the continuity of the intense staff–student as well as the student–student interactions which, from many educational viewpoints, provide necessary components of effective learning situations. Such continuity makes it possible to build rapport between staff and the students which can be useful in breaking down the inhibitions many students have in the large forum about asking questions of, or voicing their opinions to, an expert. The benefits are then transferable to resource sessions with experts from other areas either from within the wider university community or from outside agencies.

Having a limited number of staff presenting the biological and physical sciences also means that student feedback about the structure, content and intelligibility of sessions can have an immediate influence on subsequent sessions. It also makes it possible for students to receive consistent stimulation in the inquiry methods being fostered by a problem-based approach to learning.

A major concern for many beginning nursing students is the aura surrounding the 'science they will need to know' to be able to graduate as registered nurses. Many students arrive with preconceived ideas about the complexity of science, with concerns about their ability to understand, and in many instances with no idea of the relevance of science to their future nursing practice. Following are some responses from students in week one of Year 1 when asked, 'how do you feel about the science you will be doing in this course?':

> *overwhelmed; challenged; apprehensive; confused; excited; enthusiastic; scared that won't know enough at the end of the course.*

As, even today, the majority of nursing students are female, this concern about the science components of the course is compounded by widespread prejudices about girls' ability to undertake science and mathematics. There has been an ever-increasing input into primary and secondary education in the past few years as a way of actively encouraging girls into the pursuit of science, but the views long held by many that 'girls can't do science' have not yet been totally overcome.

In many traditional nursing courses students perceived much of the science content as something that had to be passed in the first year before getting on with the 'real' nursing subjects. Within an integrated problem-based learning approach, where science input is an integral component of all years of the course, a major aim is to break down these distinctions between 'real nursing' and 'science'. By approaching nursing education from a fully integrated perspective it is envisaged that there will be an acknowledgement by nursing students of the underlying importance of science knowledge, and that it will be seen to inform their practices from the beginning of their studies. By placing this integrated approach within the context of a reiterative problem-based course, the relevance of science concepts to nursing practice should be even further enhanced.

Strategies for integration

By consistently encouraging student input, the integrated nature of the course can be used to dispel the idea of science as something separate from the rest of nursing knowledge. This integration is very effectively promoted by the inclusion of scientific inquiry, principles and experiments within the nursing laboratories. A very successful example of how this occurred in a learning package incorporating issues associated with renal failure and dialysis is described in Chapter 2. A nursing laboratory designed to allow the exploration of dialysis equipment was run in conjunction with a series of simple experiments. Dialysis tubing, with various combinations of solutions of starch, iodine, copper sulphate and water, demonstrated the principles of osmosis and diffusion. A worksheet which accompanied the laboratory helped to focus student inquiry on the underlying principles and thereby enhance their understanding of the clinical implications of renal dialysis. (See Chapter 4 and Appendix 3.)

Animal dissection can also provide a valuable adjunct to student understanding. With their first introduction to the excretory system in the context of urine analysis as part of health assessment in the first year, students expressed no need to explore the intricacies of kidney anatomy. When the excretory system again surfaced within the context of kidney failure and dialysis, many students now felt the need to explore the actual details of the kidney; the opportunity to dissect a sheep kidney with models and wall charts of the human system at hand was then provided. The flexibility of the problem-based approach therefore allows the students some degree of latitude as to the depth to which they investigate a concept at each stage of their inquiry.

Similarly, within the context of several learning packages, students expressed difficulty in understanding the concept of body cavities and space, either within the healthy body or after an operation for organ removal such as hysterectomy. For some students who had never seen inside a body, a simple mouse dissection allowed them to conceptualise body space, while for others the opportunity during clinical placement to observe an operation provided this insight.

The combination of animal dissection, human models and worksheets with prompting questions can provide a very effective method for student investigation of more complex situations. Chapter 2 describes how a learning package in the final year of the course involved the students in the investigation of all the clients presenting to an accident and emergency department during one shift. This package prompted the integration of the science knowledge students had already gained from the various learning packages over the previous two years. Students were given the opportunity in the laboratory to dissect a sheep's pluck. This together with the use of human models and a series of questions arising from information relevant to two of the clients, both of whom presented to an accident and emergency department with shortness of breath as one of their symptoms, encouraged them to establish links within the respiratory and circulatory systems, and then within the whole body. (See Appendix 4.)

The reiterative nature of the course is also of major importance for building a substantial science framework on which students can base later investigations or inquiries. Each time a student meets a particular concept they should be adding to some already established knowledge base. A good example of the reiterative nature of the course lies in the examination of the concept of respiration.

Students first meet this concept early in Module 1 of Semester 1 in Year 1, where the focus is on health and wellness. They encounter respiration in the context of health assessment and explore the measurement of respiration and the underlying principles of gaseous exchange. Some students at this stage may wish to explore the concept further, but in the context of the package there is no real necessity for more in-depth inquiry, although this is never discouraged.

The next major encounter is in Semester 1 of Year 2, with a learning package developed around a client with chronic obstructive airway disease. Here students are encouraged to explore the anatomy of the respiratory tract along with the physiology of respiration; pressure changes; gaseous exchange; osmosis; a beginning understanding of blood gases; pH; acid base balance; and the patho-physiology of respiratory disorders. All of these concepts are revisited in more depth in Semester 2, Year 2 in a package focusing on cystic fibrosis; by this stage it is expected that students will have a substantial understanding of respiratory acidosis; alkalosis; arterial blood gas analysis; pH; and renal compensation. Students should be starting to recognise the intricate inter-relationships of the body systems and to realise the error of looking at any one system in isolation. They should be dealing rather with the idea that each part of body which they encounter is one component of a whole and needs to be dealt with in relation to all other components.

In Year 3 of the course the elements of respiration are addressed more fully in the clinical context of situations involving various clients as they present to an emergency department and clients in a critical care unit on mechanical ventilation. The relationships of the various body systems now take on much more meaning as clients with multi-system breakdown give the students insight into the fact that the slightest alteration to any one system of the body has ramifications for all other systems.

The reiterative nature of the course is also evidenced by the student inquiry process itself where, by the later stages of Year 1, students use their ability to draw on earlier science sessions to inform their knowledge and practice in processing the learning packages. One of the very first learning packages early in Semester 1 of Year 1 was drawn from a setting involving a school health nurse and a young adolescent, *Anthea Sharpe*, who thought she was pregnant. A few of the learning issues which some students identified during the processing of this material related to sexually transmitted diseases, the agents responsible for these diseases and the relative size of the infecting microorganisms. A science discovery laboratory focused on introductory microbiology was provided, and during this session students inoculated agar plates with their hands before and after washing with various cleansing agents; with swabs taken from benches, door handles, taps, etc; or by coughing or talking onto them. The plates were examined after a day's incubation at 37°C. For some students the relevance of what they had observed was not fully recognised until they began processing the *Timothy Randall* package towards the end of Semester 2, when they were able to use this initial laboratory to provide valuable insight into disease transmission, barrier nursing and infection control. Sexually transmitted diseases, addressed in depth by some of the students during the *Anthea Sharpe* package, had also now been specifically triggered, allowing those students who had not investigated them earlier to do so.

Similarly, the immune system, encountered in the context of infant immunisation at the beginning of Semester 2, was now revisited with *Timothy Randall* in the situation of acquired immune deficiency. Students actively drew on their knowledge of the healthy immune system to initiate their investigations into the compromised system. This reiterative capacity needs to be exploited both in the design of the curriculum and in the facilitation of student learning.

Because of the more self-directed nature of Year 3 of the course, students in small groups or as a whole-year student body can request science sessions to address particular issues arising from the packages they are processing or areas where they lack knowledge. They may also, particularly in small-group tutorials, ask staff to review various concepts already encountered during the course to date, but which they feel some need to cover again with assistance from a specialised science facilitator. Comments from Year 3 students support the use of the smaller tutorial format.

> We used to have large group science lectures; however in third year small-group science was much more effective.
>
> *Group 4, Year 3*

By Year 3 of the course the integrated nature of the learning is more apparent: students tend not to identify specifically scientific issues as required learning needs but rather to generalise a learning issue which may have a science focus as one component. Students soon recognise that resource sessions dedicated to science components are not the only way in which to gain access to scientific knowledge and feel more comfortable with raising science issues in a variety of forums.

As the course is constantly trying to eliminate fragmenting distinctions between science and other nursing knowledge, both staff and students may lose sight of the necessity to be continually questioning the level of understanding of the underlying scientific principles. Proficiency in science content needs to be adequately addressed if students are to develop a holistic approach to their professional practice. To this end the majority of assessment items set for students should contain some element of science, and this should be clearly identified in the assessment criteria so that students continue to be aware of the importance of science in their understanding of nursing.

Is there a need for additional strategies?

One problem frequently voiced by students, particularly in the early stages of entering a problem-based course, is that they don't know what they need to know. They may feel so overwhelmed by a particular topic that they express difficulty in identifying specific learning issues and particularly are unable to formulate questions for science resource sessions. If this happens it is essential that the science expert is not working in isolation from the rest of the teaching team. There is a need for consultation and co-operation between all the facilitators in order to respond adequately. The primary outcome of the problem-based tutorials should be the processing of information in such a manner that students are able to identify specific learning issues. The investigation of these gaps in knowledge is then the primary responsibility of the student group, either as individuals giving feedback to the whole group or as a smaller sub-group, again giving feedback. By the end of a problem-based tutorial it is essential that students have:

- articulated what they need to learn following the problem-based tutorial (in order to make progress with their inquiry – proving of hypotheses, etc.)
- established clearly how they will organise themselves to do this learning and how and when they will (where relevant) share it with the group.

The facilitator's guiding role is vital to ensure that student articulation of what they need to learn is tending in the right direction. It is after feedback sessions that difficulties in understanding particular concepts may warrant the need for expert resource sessions. It may still be difficult for students to formulate questions about these learning issues; these may be addressed in the initial phase of the course by asking students not necessarily to provide questions for resource sessions, but rather to supply lists of words, phrases, ideas or statements which they have encountered or identified during the processing of the package and which require some further clarification.

Difficulty in processing the learning issues identified during the problem-based tutorials to a point where it is obvious that expert input is required is often compounded by constraints on timetabling and room availability. In Year 1 of the course at Griffith University this meant that the science fixed-resource sessions normally had to be held on the morning immediately after students first encountered a new learning package. This allowed very little time for processing of material and integration of pre-existing knowledge with newly sought knowledge, and it resulted in minimal input by students prior to the science sessions. Where this time constraint can be overcome a more valuable student-directed session is possible.

Science resource sessions in a course such as this can take on many forms. In the first two years, the sessions are primarily designed for the participation of the whole year group. They may encompass a quasi lecture format; question-answer sessions with either student-directed or faculty-directed questions; laboratory sessions either within the nominal nursing laboratory time or in the scheduled fixed-resource time – space permitting; viewing of appropriate videos; animal or tissue dissections; or any other activity which encourages student enquiry.

There will be the necessity at times for explanatory sessions where the expert has major input into the discussions. These normally arise if a large number of students or several of the groups have identified a similar learning need. For example, in the first semester of the course students met the concept of blood pressure for the first time during their investigations into health assessment and the whole student group recognised the need to know how to measure blood pressure. This was addressed in their nursing laboratory time, but a large group of students also wanted extra input in order to understand adequately the scientific principles behind blood pressure so that they could correctly interpret the measurements they would make. This need for understanding the underlying principles was also very clearly established when one student asked during a science fixed-resource session:

> *I went to a doctor recently for a medical examination and was told that my blood pressure was normal. How could I have blood pressure, I'm not sick?*
>
> *Rebecca, Year 1 student*

This question, along with others submitted before the session, worked as a trigger for an explanatory resource session dealing with the principles of physics underlying pressure in fluids and movement of fluids, as well as an introduction to the circulatory system.

Another instance in which expert explanations or discussion for the whole class may be appropriate is in the first use of a developed learning package when what was thought of by the faculty as relevant and necessary science knowledge has not been adequately triggered by the provided materials. Students may therefore not have initiated any enquiry into these science aspects and so have not generated any learning issues or questions. This situation may arise not only because of lack of adequate trigger material but also through inadequate facilitation within the problem-based tutorial (see Chapter 3 on facilitation for further discussion of this aspect). Once again it is essential for there to be co-operation with the science resource faculty in the preparatory stages of learning packages and in the compilation of facilitator guides for use with these packages (see Chapter 2). If the situation has arisen because of inadequate trigger material, this can be corrected by the addition of suitable stimulus material for subsequent running of the package when appropriate evaluation procedures have been used to examine all aspects of course design. The importance of systematic feedback and review cannot be over-stressed.

The most successful resource sessions, from the faculty perspective, are those which are student-driven or directed, preferably by student questions submitted to the resource person a reasonable time before the session or else as questions from the floor during the session. This situation tends to place the resource person in the unenviable position of the 'expert'. Although this may be quite appropriate for a clinical nurse specialist who has been brought in to address an area of exper-tise with which she/he works daily, for the science resource person this is often not the case and they may have a need for prior reading and research. In this position the resource person must be open in admitting gaps in their knowledge; not be afraid of making mistakes and having students query them; and not hesitate to correct mis-information at a later date.

The sessions which run as open questions from the floor do present an ideal situation for reinforcing the concept of knowledge already existing among students, particularly if students are actively encouraged to share knowledge in this larger forum. Students themselves, however, often believe their questions to be too trivial and fear the ridicule of their peers if they voice their queries or express their opinions in front of the large group. As group learning and group process develop during the course, the willingness of students to speak up in the large forum does increase. This type of interaction must be continually and consistently encouraged from the outset and students must be reassured of the validity of their inquiries, no matter how naive they may appear.

The situation where student questions are submitted well before a scheduled session allows the resource person to come armed with the knowledge not only to answer the specific questions but also to extend the inquiry. It also permits the dissemination of knowledge to students in a context, in this case clinical, which validates the necessity for them to acquire it.

> *Our problem-based learning method is the closest thing you can get to the clinical situation of caring for clients.*
>
> *Esther, Year 3 student*

As the students progress through the three years of the course it is possible to see an evolution with respect to their questions and identified learning issues. This often gives an indication of the difficulty students have in gaining access to infor-mation. Where do they go to look? So many of the texts are not designed for use in any way but by working from A to B to C, and a problem-based learning approach by no means follows such a formula. If, for example, their query was in a package one of the aspects of which was immunity, and they came across a mention of 'B and T cells', many students at the beginning of the course would have no idea where to go to find the necessary information. We must stress again that teaching, i.e. the facilitation of learning, cannot sensibly be reduced to 'content' knowledge. It also involves 'how to function' in the area of study, including where and how to seek needed information. In the first year this will include the elementary 'where and how do I look', and will become more sophisticated in later years. It is imperative that facilitators are able to give guidance to students on background reading for specific topics so that questions can be generated before they attend resource sessions.

Some examples of questions and issues submitted by students before fixed resource sessions are included here to indicate the developmental nature of this process.

Year 1 – Semester 1 – Health and Wellness – 'microbiology of hand washing – How long do you wash your hands?' 'T and B cells'

Year 1 – Semester 2 – Timothy Randall package – 'What is the actual difference between HIV and AIDS?'

These questions mostly indicate a difficulty on the students' part in knowing where to gain access to the necessary information, as the answers to these queries are all readily available from various written sources.

Year 2 – Semester 2 – Bruce Wayne package – 'Would Intracranial Pressure increase when there is a deficit in kidney/renal function resulting in Central Nervous System complications i.e. seizures?'

Jack Foster (Alcohol dependence package) – 'Why is a person hungry/thirsty during a hangover?'

Questions by this stage in Year 2 are generally more to do with a difficulty in relating knowledge from different areas rather than with not knowing where to look. This is not to say that Year 2 students are no longer trying to get the 'expert' or their facilitator to tell them all they need to know, but this is not happening all the time and they are taking more responsibility for their learning.

Year 3 – Semester 2 – questions submitted to visiting palliative care specialist on pain. 'How do health care professionals know how much

> *pain relief to give? What forms of assessment/indications do you use? How do they know where the line between pain management and euthanasia is?'*

These questions are obviously interdisciplinary and again have to do with the integration of information which is not readily available in texts or journal articles. A comment from a Year 3 student at the end of the course reflects the success of this process.

> *The fact that you work from the problem makes the comprehension of integrating all the different issues together a lot clearer. I have also become more aware of where to find knowledge and the links between issues from learning in this manner.*
>
> *Hue, Year 3 student*

It is essential for the resource person to go to a resource session prepared to explain in a variety of ways and to be flexible enough to move with the requirements of the large group. If nothing has been submitted before a session and students are unwilling to ask any questions at the outset, another useful strategy is to begin the session by eliciting some information of a general nature from individuals within the group on a specific component which you, as the 'expert', have identified as a significant learning issue. For example, the first science resource session for a learning package involving an elderly woman presenting signs of dementia was started by asking for individual students to share with the large group any definition of dementia that they had located in the literature. These were listed on the whiteboard and augmented with any alternative ones from the resource person. The students, as individuals, were then asked to determine any similarities and/or differences within these definitions, and this served as a basis to start discussion on the underlying concepts of dementia in the context of the particular problem situation under investigation. Variations on this strategy could involve subdividing the larger student body into smaller groups to undertake the initial compilation of the different definitions; small group discussion on similarities and differences to synthesise an overarching definition for presentation back to the whole student body; or any of a variety of approaches which could stimulate more student participation.

Where does this leave fixed-resource sessions?

Provided that fixed-resource sessions can be structured and run in accordance with the learning principles embodied in problem-based learning, there are several roles for them within an integrated problem-based learning course. These lie, essentially, in providing: a forum for discussion between the student body and an expert or experts in a particular field; an arena for the dissemination of information or knowledge and the discussion of the unpublished results of recent pertinent research; an occasion for an explanation of difficult content or concepts; and, most importantly, an opportunity for the encouragement of students to investigate further their understanding of a specific topic.

The fixed-resource session can take on one of many formats depending on the route of enquiry anticipated by the faculty preparing the learning package. In many instances, the session may be most successfully facilitated by a clinical nurse specialist from the particular area. During Year 2 of the course health breakdown becomes a major focus and in a learning package incorporating concepts related to cardiovascular disease, the information about the recording, use and interpretation of electrocardiograms is most effectively conveyed by someone dealing with this technology on a daily basis. Specialists from other discipline areas also serve to give the students a much wider outlook into the necessary understanding they require of a particular situation in order to make informed clinical judgements. Both a pharmacist associated with a hospital respiratory ward and a naturopath using an alternative approach to treatment were used as resource people during a learning package which involved a child with cystic fibrosis. Legal experts with either a nursing or a purely legal background were used to provide students with an insight into the legal responsibilities of the nursing profession within some of the learning packages. Members of community help or support groups also provide a valuable resource pool for informing the student body of these essential adjuncts to the holistic treatment of their future clients.

Within the limited time scales of a university course, it is often a very successful strategy to present a session with a panel of experts or lay people involved in a particular area. In dealing with a learning package where the client was diagnosed with Parkinson's disease, a panel consisting of a clinical nurse consultant on continence, a volunteer from the Parkinson's self-help group and a nurse from a rehabilitation unit provided the students with a cross-section of people directly involved with clients who have Parkinson's disease; they could direct questions raised during their investigations into the disorder to these people. Often panels can be formed from within the teaching faculty. For example, when dealing with childbirth, qualified midwives on the school staff can provide the panel members; in the case of mental health investigations, faculty qualified in the area of psychiatric nursing can form a resource panel. This strategy also conveys to the students the expert knowledge contained within the school and reinforces the often overlooked fact that the majority of the teaching staff are registered nurses.

Assessment

Feedback from students across the three years of this course at Griffith University to date has indicated that they believed not enough emphasis has been placed on the assessment of their science understanding. They admitted the importance of understanding the science but tended to put this to one side if assessment items did not require an explicit science component. This problem has been addressed to some extent, particularly in the third year of the course where assessment items were designed which more specifically required the student to address science as an integral component of their assessment discussion. An essay topic used as part of individual assessment for the clinical placements in semester 3 of Year 3 is given in Figure 4.1.

One of the major assessment areas in which an indication of the depth of the students' knowledge base with respect to scientific principles can readily be determined is in the Global Nursing Practice Assessment (GNPA). Either through judicious questioning of the student during or after the client interaction or via a written discussion paper concentrating on the linking of science concepts to the specific client situation, a clear indication of the ability of the student to incorporate science principles into practice can be obtained.

Another example of strategies for encouraging students to ascertain their own level of understanding of particular concepts lies in the use of worksheets. As one aim of the course is to encourage self-directedness, self-assessment or formative assessment in the guise of worksheets which students can use as they wish can

---

Pertinent criteria were used to draw the student's attention to ways of incorporating science principles; for example:

- Discusses the complexity of the client situation by discussing more than one body system and an understanding of social, political, economic and emotional issues.

- Discussion reflects a holistic approach to nursing practice relating to a specific client situation.

From your current clinical placement select a client with complex health-breakdown involving more than one body system. The chosen client will be someone with whom you are actively involved and who prompts you to identify Situations in Need of Improvement (SINIs). Describe the client situation in detail identifying your hypotheses and your clinical judgements. Discuss the learning issues which informed your clinical decision-making process. Critically reflect on and evaluate your intervention and its effectiveness.

Figure 4.1: Essay 2500–3000 words

provide a valuable adjunct to student learning. Within the reiterative framework of the course, worksheets which prompt students to check their knowledge before they move onto a more complex investigation of any particular area can play an important role. There can therefore be an expectation that students will attend fixed-resource sessions with a certain level of understanding, and the onus is then placed on the student to initiate questioning of the resource person if there is a deficit in it. (See Appendix 5.)

The flexibility of the course also encourages students to seek extra help when faced with particular difficulties. As many of our students may have been away from an educational institution for many years or may have had no formal education in science, there is often a perceived need by these students for extra science sessions to cover basic material assumed as common knowledge by all school leavers. These issues are most effectively addressed in small group tutorials where students feel less inhibited and are free to ask even the most basic questions. Within this course, the students are told at the beginning of each year that such science small groups are possible, but it is up to them to initiate the process; this once again encourages them to take the responsibility for their own learning.

Conclusion

Some of the many and varied ways in which knowledges can be integrated into a problem-based curriculum have been introduced in this chapter by discussing the experience of science integration into a nursing course. It is shown how such an integration can enrich student learning and allow them to integrate their own knowledge and experience within a wide range of possible learning situations.

Chapter 5
Integrating knowledges in the laboratory

Jan Cattoni

> *Our problem-based learning method is the closest thing you can get to the clinical situation of caring for clients.*
>
> *Tyrone, student*

In this chapter we examine the place of laboratories in a problem-based course. The chapter traces the history of the development of laboratories in this programme, and will provide a number of different laboratory designs that were developed to meet student learning needs. The laboratories relate to two specific learning packages, *Timothy Randall* and *Bruce Wayne*, outlined in Chapters 1 and 2 respectively. The first learning package dealt with a young man's experience of discovering his own HIV status and later coping with his partner's death. The *Bruce Wayne* package focused on a child receiving peritoneal dialysis for chronic renal failure and on his parent's perspective whilst he was awaiting a donor kidney. *Timothy Randall* laboratories provide an example of how laboratories can be used creatively to meet specific student learning needs. *Bruce Wayne* laboratories will demonstrate how science concepts can be integrated and assessed in the laboratory setting. The range of laboratories presented should convey a sense of the capacity for flexibility and creativity that laboratory design can provide.

History of laboratories in the programme

When the programme was first established we had not fully thought through the idea of laboratories or the form they might take. Much energy had been devoted to writing learning packages and identifying expert people who could provide fixed-resource sessions. We had a fully equipped simulated thirty-bed ward area that was available for students' use. In addition we had a fully equipped wet lab for science experiments and dissections. We organised a number of semi-structured laboratories for Semester 1 for students to learn some basic health assessment skills. In Semester 2, however, as students moved from a health focus to areas of health breakdown and individual adaptation and loss, it became evident that some learning issues required a different learning environment to facilitate learning. For example, the questions: *How will I know that I will be able to function as a nurse in such situations?* and *How will I cope when I have to deal with people in situations like this?* emerged often.

As students began to go out on clinical placements, similar questions began to surface from the clinical agencies who asked: *How will we know what your students can competently do in the clinical setting?* and *In what instances will they need supervision?* These questions raised two separate but related sets of issues.

Many agencies were used to a nurse education system where discrete nursing practices were identified by the educational institution and usually placed within a separate course that might be called something like 'Clinical Competencies'. Often these competencies were limited to psychomotor skills – for example, taking blood pressures and doing wound dressings – and were divided across the three years of a course according to notions of the complexity of the skill. A Year 1 student, for example, might be identified as someone who could do X number of simple skills in contrast to a Year 3 student who presumably could do three times as many of the more complex skills. (This is a hangover from the apprenticeship training system and from the military dynamics of nursing organisation that supported the apprenticeship system.)

One of the main difficulties with this approach is that it privileged psychomotor skills over other less tangible skills such as counselling and time management, and also created a hierarchy of skills. That is, some skills such as inserting an indwelling catheter into the bladder were seen as much more important than others, as only more senior persons were allowed to practise them. Other skills, such as attending to personal hygiene and skin integrity, were seen as less important skills – in spite of their capacity to influence a patient's state of comfort – because more junior staff were allowed to attend to them. Furthermore, by focusing on skills in a de-contextualised manner the whole issue of the patient and their experience of their situation was de-emphasised.

Our organisation of course material attempted to break up the skills hierarchy by introducing clients with a wide range of problems incorporating in any one semester a variety of nursing practices from the simple to the complex (see Figure 5.1). The trigger material and the accompanying laboratories attempted to place communication and people-focused skills on an equal, and in some instances more important footing than psychomotor skills. At the same time we acknowledged that patients had a right to expect that those caring for them were sufficiently competent to provide safe and effective care.

Figure 5.1 shows a proforma that was developed for the clinical agencies in response to some of their questions. As a team we identified skills we believed

Modular focus (concepts)	Week	Learning package	Nursing practices & issues covered in labs	On-campus assessment required	Related nursing practices that can be undertaken in the clinical area
Module 1 Nursing and Adaptation	1 & 2	LP1 Kathy Peters and Lal Nguyan (cultural differences and the birthing experience)	Baby bathing, Baby assessment, Introduction to discharge planning, Post-natal assessment	No	Students can continue to develop these skills in the relevant clinical setting with appropriate supervision. Baby bathing, Baby assessment, Post-natal assessment
	3	**Clinical placement 1**			
	4 & 5	LP2 Greg Stone (young man diagnosed schizophrenic)	Introduction to mental illness concepts, Extended communication skills, Intra-muscular injections, Legal aspects of drug administration, Anatomy and physiology	Yes	Informed consent IMI administration, Effects of drugs and client/nurse responses to IMI, Investigation of pharmacological substances
	6	**Clinical placement 2**			
	7 & 8	LP3 The Heridan Family (gastro enteritis hospitalisation)	Fluid balance concepts, Infection control, Dealing with infected waste	No	Fluid balance assessment and recording, Paediatric assessment, Barrier nursing

Module	Week	Lecture/Topic	Lab	Lab content
Module 2 Nursing and the Experience of Loss	9	LP1	Wound dressing Removal of drain/sutures Altered body image Psychological impact of change Client teaching	Yes	Simple wound dressings Removal of sutures Removal of drains Communication with clients under-going alterations in body image
	10	**Clinical placement 3**		
	11	Sarah Henderson (postmastectomy) contd		
	12 & 13	LP2 Tim Randall (HIV)	Introduction to AIDS Death Last offices Disposal of infected waste products Confidentiality Communication with grieving relatives Guided imagery	No	Handling of infectious materials Care of the dead body Communication with grieving persons
	14	Course Enrichment Week	Assessment of aseptic technique Client teaching and communication		
	15	**Clinical placement 4**		
	16	LP3 Mr Walker (occupational health, glaucoma and early retirement)	No lab	No	Introduction to occupational health Psychological impact of health-related redundancy

Figure 5.1: Overview of Semester 2

should be assessed before they were practised on real people. We identified skills – such as administering drugs – that had the potential to compromise a patient's health if carried out incorrectly as skills which needed to be assessed on-campus. The proforma also identified the areas that students had covered in laboratories and those skills students could practise with supervision. This document met the needs of the clinical area and enabled agency staff to see just where students were in relation to their learning.

If we consider the student questions at the beginning of this chapter, how do we meet these students' learning needs? Let us return to Timothy Randall's situation which was explored in Chapter 1. In this learning package the nurse is required to function in a number of contexts. Initially she is required to support Colin and Timothy following the disclosure of Timothy's HIV status. Later in the package she is required both to care for Colin, who is dying, and to support his loved ones upon his death. During the problem-based tutorials students researched much of the knowledge they would need to possess in fulfilling their nursing roles; however, they were concerned with how they would actually perform and cope in such situations and variations of such situations in practice.

The fairly prescriptive structure for skills teaching in the nursing laboratory inherited from previous models of nursing education did not sit comfortably with a problem-based philosophy. In most hospital training settings and in many university settings, simulated wards peopled with plastic dummies are the main environment for students to simulate practice before going into clinical settings and performing skills on real people. The role of the teacher in this approach is to demonstrate how a skill is performed with the student observing and then attempting to perform the skill.

In relation to *Timothy Randall*'s situation, the traditional approach might recognise discrete skills such as *barrier nursing* (nursing practices that protect the nurse while caring for someone with an infectious disease) and *laying out the dead* (care of the body after death) among the list of easily identified and traditionally accepted nursing skills that students are expected to master and that a teacher could demonstrate. Students would also be taught the theories behind barrier nursing in the classroom. In the case of barrier nursing this would include some theory on microbiology and cross-infection. Students would then practise under supervision in the simulated setting. At a later stage, students might then be formally assessed on how well they carry out the task according to a formula for that task's mastery. They would then be allowed to apply the formula to situations they encountered in the clinical setting. Often the formal assessment would be carried out on a plastic dummy in the simulated ward setting. As a team we felt this approach was not in keeping with a problem-based course and was inappropriate for student learning generally.

What was omitted when psychomotor skills were privileged in situations like Timothy's were practices such as values clarification, grief counselling and client advocacy that were less tangible but equally important in the provision of effective care. The patient was also relegated to the status of a non-feeling, non-speaking being. There was little scope for students to test their knowledge-base in situations where the formula might need to be adapted; and, more importantly, there was no space for the students to explore their own feelings and fears in relation to such situations. These issues seemed to be central to the questions students themselves were posing. With their input we developed two laboratories to assist them in meeting their learning needs.

The *Timothy Randall* laboratories

The two laboratories accompanying this learning package were designed to address two main learning areas that students themselves had identified. The first related to how students would cope with issues raised by the package such as death and caring for dying persons and their families. The package prompted many issues from the students' own experiences. Many of them were reminded of painful experiences related to the death of friends and family and many tutorials found students in tears, with other group members displaying a range of responses to the situation. Some students were angry that the process was proving very painful, some were awkward and others found a need to talk about their experiences.

This seemed an important opportunity for students to explore and reflect upon their own responses to death and to begin to feel comfortable with the responses of others. We believed it was important that students develop skills in self-awareness and self-care in order to cope with and survive the situations they would encounter as registered nurses.

It is worth pointing out that many facilitators also found themselves confronted with unresolved issues relating to death in their own lives. It was important to identify this for staff before the start of the learning package and to provide support for each other while the package was running. Many facilitators needed support in order to facilitate student learning in these very difficult circumstances. The willingness to express sadness and obtain support from each other operated as a parallel to the students' experiences.

In the first laboratory students were asked to form in groups of ten and wear comfortable clothing. Students arrived to a darkened quiet room, lay down on mattresses, were shown a number of relaxation exercises and were taken through some guided imagery by the facilitator. The imagery, which is outlined below, involved the life cycle of a flower and lasted approximately twenty minutes.

*Students arrive for this laboratory and lie down in a quiet darkened room on mattresses on the floor.
*The facilitator guides the students through a standard set of relaxation exercises then begins the following:

> I'd like you to imagine you are a flower in the bush. Become this flower. Visualise yourself and your surroundings ... take some time to get the feeling of being a flower ... what kind of flower are you? What kind of leaves and petals do you have ... what kind of things happen to you as this flower? Feel the sun on your petals (Breeze, rain, dew ...)
>
> Someone comes to look at you. What is the attitude to this visitor? Now become the visitor looking at yourself – what do you see – what feelings do you have?
>
> Now become the flower again ... the sun is disappearing, the night is becoming cold – the first frosts touch your petals – be aware of yourself as the flower – how do you feel? Your petals are turning brown and starting to wither, your stem is starting to wilt – be aware of your feelings – do you notice anything about yourself you did not notice before? ... It is now very dark and cold and you know that you will not survive the night ... as cold numbs you become aware that you can leave something of yourself behind after your death – what will you leave behind? Become whatever you leave behind – what are you like? What are your characteristics?
>
> Now become your self again and slowly say goodbye to the bush, to the flower and whatever you have left behind ... rest quietly for a little while.

*Afterwards students were encouraged to share their thoughts on the imagery and then relate these thoughts to their feelings about death. The depth of disclosure and discussion was determined by the students themselves with the facilitator merely providing some trigger questions. Some examples are shown below.
*The facilitator then talks with the students about their responses to the imagery. This exercise needs a delicate debrief as students are commonly quite distressed.

Figure 5.2:   Guided imagery laboratory

There was a significant degree of variation from one group's responses to the next to this experience. Most groups were able to make connections between their own responses to death and their responses to Timothy and Colin's situation. For many students this was an important discovery as it enabled them to recognise that they engaged with the patient situation to a far greater extent than they might have expected. Facilitators made themselves available to students after these sessions to provide support as the need arose. Many students took advantage of this opportunity, particularly if they had felt unable to talk during the session. In some instances students were referred to the student counsellor. Figure 5.3 gives examples of trigger questions facilitators used to help students process their experiences in this laboratory.

*Can you talk about the kind of flower you chose to be? Can you describe it?
*How did you feel about the visitor?
*What did you see when you became the visitor?
*How did you feel when night fell and you knew you were going to die?
*What did you choose to leave behind?
*Were there other issues that came to mind during the imagery?
*Is there any unfinished business?

Figure 5.3: Trigger questions

The second laboratory was held in the simulated ward area and students again formed groups of eight to ten. This laboratory was designed to address students' concerns about how they might function as nurses in the given situation. This laboratory also enabled students to apply science concepts such as cross-infection that they had visited earlier in the semester. Students were presented ahead of time with a number of scenarios to work through. This enabled them to research their learning issues and come prepared for the laboratory. They were encouraged to do their research in groups. The scenarios placed the students in the role of the registered nurse and involved Timothy and Colin.

The scenarios were developed in consultation with actual patients and nurses working in the clinical area and were chosen as situations that represented typical issues in the area of HIV/AIDS care. There was significant input from the science staff member to ensure that the scenarios provided sufficient scope for students to apply science concepts. A specialist registered nurse working in the area of HIV/AIDS care was available to the students during the laboratory to answer questions and provide guidance. This was of particular use to students as they were able to obtain answers to the questions that emerged as a result of working through the scenarios. The responses that the specialist nurse was able to provide resulted from her own expertise and familiarity with the most up-to-date medical knowledge in this field. The students also had a facilitator available to each group. Below is an example of the laboratory sheets provided ahead of time for students to allow them to undertake the necessary research.

Section A

1. Meet with your group and facilitator and discuss the plans and ideas that you have for the scenarios. Identify learning issues and available resources and research these before the laboratory.

2. Upon arrival in the laboratory organise yourself around a bed area. Identify group members to role-play Timothy, Colin and the nurse for each scenario. Video playback facilities are available for your use.

3. When you have worked through the scenarios view the video with your facilitator. Evaluate how the group worked through the scenarios. Identify outstanding learning issues.

Section B

Scenario 1. You are asked to take a phone inquiry regarding Colin. A man identifies himself as Colin's friend and tells you that he has just heard that Colin is ill. He asks you how he is and what is wrong with him.

Scenario 2. Colin buzzes on the nurse call bell. You enter his room and find him very distressed. He has been trying to peel an orange and has cut the palm of his hand quite deeply. There is blood on Colin's clothes, the bedside table and the knife. He looks like he will need sutures.

Scenario 3. Colin has been febrile and sweating profusely. You offer to provide a bed sponge which he accepts.

Scenario 4. Colin has just died. As his primary carer you are required to lay out his body. Timothy asks if he can assist you.

Figure 5.4:   Timothy Randall laboratory sheet

The necessary props were also available in the laboratory. These constituted all the equipment a student would be likely to encounter in the clinical setting, such as a range of disinfecting substances, telephones and extensions, suture sets, body bags, etc. The availability of *real* equipment enabled the students to familiarise themselves with these objects without the stress of having to function in the actual situation. Using the knowledge obtained before the laboratory the students were required to make a number of decisions in each scenario. Students were also encouraged to role-play the patient and the nurse for each scenario and rotate these roles for each scenario. This ensured that the patient was represented as a real person, and it enabled all students to explore the roles. Texts were also available for the students to use during the laboratory itself.

In the first situation students had to decide what information would be appropriate to tell Colin's friend. Theoretically they were all very conscious of confidentiality issues and had decided what information should be given. Using phone lines set up in the ward, students found it difficult to limit themselves to this information when the caller was particularly assertive or distressed. After considerable discussion the students were able to develop effective strategies for dealing with such situations. These included identifying, in consultation with Timothy and Colin, a family member who was prepared to receive calls inquiring about Colin. Similarly in the second scenario, students had to prioritise tasks, integrating knowledge on cross-infection, haemorrhage, shock, and wound care.

In this scenario the use of video playback was particularly effective. Students were often able to identify problems immediately with their actions. Given the complexity of the scenario students had to select priorities for their actions. For example, should they stop the bleeding first, or put gloves on? What actions should they take to alleviate the bleeding? How might the student react to the sight of Colin's blood, and will this influence how Colin feels? Students in role as the patient were also able to provide feedback on their perceptions from the perspective of the patient. The facilitator can challenge the students on the basis of their decisions or provide the students with variations of the scenario to enable them to test their understanding more comprehensively.

The Bruce Wayne laboratories

Another example of a series of laboratories that worked to extrapolate many learning issues for students were the laboratories accompanying the *Bruce Wayne* learning package. As you may recall from Chapter 2, *Bruce Wayne* was an 8-year-old boy with chronic renal failure. In the package, students first meet him in the emergency department following a seizure at home. In subsequent blocks of material students are required to manage peritoneal dialysis in an intensive care setting and later deal with a situation where the dialysis becomes disconnected. Full details of the block material are contained in Chapter 2. The laboratories developed to accompany this package were designed to help students gain confidence in the practice setting.

The first laboratory provided the students with their second opportunity to explore neurological status. Even though the primary physiological focus in the learning package was the renal system, the first block required students to explore the connections between different body systems. Students had access to *Bruce Wayne*'s case notes when he presented in the emergency department where they could have hypothesised about this underlying renal pathology. This enabled them to investigate the links between the renal system and the neurological system. The laboratory helped students understand *Bruce Wayne*'s presenting situation and enabled them to develop neurological assessment skills. Outlined in Figure 5.5 is the laboratory sheet that students received. Below each box is an explanation for that step.

Steps 1 & 2 are to be worked through before your arrival in the laboratory.

Step 1

Bruce Wayne has just arrived in the casualty department with a history of having had two 'fits' this morning. Bruce is drowsy but rousable and his status is describes as 'post-ictal'.

Below are some prompts to help you process this information.

a)   What information do you need to assess Bruce's situation?
b)   Where might you obtain this information?
c)   What equipment/skills do you need?
d)   What does this information tell us? What purposes/outcomes can it be put to?
e)   What are your responsibilities as a nurse in this situation?

Organise yourself in a group of 8–10 and work through this situation before arrival in the laboratory.

By including a scenario from the learning package, a context for skills learning is established from the outset. The set of questions that follows encourages students to direct their line of enquiry from the point of view of the nurse in the situation. This provides them with a sense of their own professional role and of the sort of expectations that will accompany that role. This step also places the responsibility for researching learning issues with the students.

Step 2

Attached is a list of trigger questions to evaluate your understanding of neurological assessment prior to arrival in the laboratory.

The trigger questions are included to enable students to evaluate their research findings before they arrive in the laboratory. They provide students with an

a) What are the factors that can contribute to a person having altered neurological status?
b) What are the signs of altered neurological status?
c) What are the different types of seizures?
d) What signs do you observe in order to identify and describe seizures?
e) What is a Glasgow Coma Scale?
f) How is it adapted for use with children and infants?
g) What is raised intracranial pressure and how do you observe for it?
h) What is the role of pupil changes in neurological status?
i) What are the cranial nerves?
j) What are the nursing responsibilities for a patient with altered neurological status?

Develop any further trigger questions from your own research below.
*
*
*
*

indication of the level of understanding they will be assumed to have before undertaking the laboratory and they act as a 'safety net' in case their self-directed research has taken them off track.

Step 3 Available Laboratory Time – 90 minutes

On arrival in the laboratory collect a neurological assessment sheet and organise yourself in pairs around a bed area.

Collect the equipment you will need to conduct your assessment from the central laboratory area.

Undertake a neurological assessment on each other utilising the neurological assessment sheet.

Write a short summary of the person's neurological status.

Discuss your summary with the facilitator available to you in the laboratory.

Are there outstanding learning issues? If so, organise a time to return to the laboratory and conduct another assessment after additional research.

This step allows the students to apply their understanding of neurological assessment in a context similar to the clinical setting. The process of selecting the equipment, undertaking the assessment, recording their findings and reporting these findings, mirrors that of the clinical setting.

Step 4

During your problem-based tutorial following the laboratory, reflect upon the following:

What do you think are the issues for a person experiencing altered neurological status?

   * for the patient?
   * for the nurse?
   * for the significant others?

What actions can you as a nurse take to support the person experiencing altered neurological status?

How will the knowledge you have gained in working through this laboratory assist you in dealing with situations like *Bruce Wayne's?*

Figure 5.5:   Neurological assessment laboratory sheet

This step enables the students to reflect on their learning experiences in the laboratory and also relate their understanding back to the learning package. It also allows the facilitator to evaluate the students' understanding of relevant concepts.

This laboratory was timetabled after students received the first block of material for the *Bruce Wayne* learning package. The laboratory design incorporated important elements of self-direction and self-evaluation. Students were encouraged to investigate learning issues and test their understanding before arrival in the laboratory. Students could then begin to integrate their understanding into the neurological assessment they were undertaking. They were then able to record their findings on neurological assessment forms similar to those found in the clinical settings and then to validate their findings with the facilitator available to them in the laboratory. This laboratory provided an introduction to neurological assessment; however, it drew on concepts visited in an earlier learning package based on a young man with a diagnosis of schizophrenia. In this earlier package students had touched on the neurological system as it pertained to this young man's situation.

In contrast, the next laboratory in the *Bruce Wayne* learning package drew on science concepts that students had dealt with on a number of occasions in the course. This is consistent with the reiterative nature of the course. The second laboratory encouraged students to explore and apply more complex science concepts, and required students to move through five separate steps which we will outline in brief in Figure 5.6. Steps 2 and 3 are outlined in more detail in Appendix 3.

Step 1

On the basis of Block 2 of *Bruce Wayne*'s learning package consider the following:

23–12–93 2230 hrs

You are about to start your shift in the paediatric Intensive Therapy Unit where you will be providing nursing care for *Bruce Wayne* who has just begun peritoneal dialysis.

Consider the following:

a) What information will you need to assess Bruce's situation and function in your role as a nurse?
b) How will you obtain this information?
c) What skills/equipment will you need?
d) What documentation will you need?
e) What are your responsibilities as a nurse caring for Bruce?

Step 2

Step 2 for this laboratory is the same as for the previous *Bruce Wayne* laboratory. In addition, students are required to have an understanding of specific science concepts relevant to the laboratory. These science concepts, which include osmosis, diffusion, etc., are outlined in full in the worksheet in Appendix 3.

Step 3

Step 3 for this laboratory was a dialysis experiment with beakers, tubing and solutions to explore the principles of dialysis as they apply to both peritoneal dialysis and haemodialysis. Students worked in groups of eight around work benches in the wet laboratory. A set of trigger questions requiring students to apply their understanding of relevant concepts accompanied the experiment. The experiment and trigger questions are also outlined in Appendix 3.

Step 4

Students move to the simulated ward from the wet laboratory

In your group examine the equipment supplied for peritoneal dialysis. Organise yourself as a group to:

1. Check the medical orders for the dialysate and additives; and for the timing of in/dwell/out phases.

2. Prime the equipment and commence the dialysis. Aprons are provided to enable you to simulate a client receiving peritoneal dialysis.

3. Document your observations during the procedure. Discuss your expectations in relation to:

   − discomfort during the procedure
   − appearance of the returned dialysate
   − running totals of amount in, out, and difference.

4. What comparisons can you draw between the experiment and peritoneal dialysis?

Step 5

During your problem-based tutorial following the laboratory reflect upon the following:

Identify where your care for Bruce may differ from the needs of an adult beginning peritoneal dialysis.

*What factors contribute to a person's developing renal failure?
*What are the differences between haemodialysis and peritoneal dialysis?
*Compare the advantages and disadvantages of both types of dialysis.
*Identify the impact of renal failure on other systems of the body.
*Identify the impact of dialysis on the family and wider social functions.
*Begin to reflect on issues relating to organ donation.

How will the knowledge you have gained in working through this laboratory assist you in dealing with situations like *Bruce Wayne's*?

Figure 5.6:   Peritoneal dialysis laboratory

Credentialling in the laboratory

The laboratory structure we have developed lends itself readily to a model for skills credentialling. At the beginning of the chapter we spoke of identifying the skills students needed to be assessed or 'credentialled' to perform before practising them on patients in the clinical setting. Examples of the skills requiring assessment are vital signs assessment, medication administration, aseptic technique and fluid management. These were seen as 'cornerstone' skills with many other skills being derived from them.

We felt it important that students were deemed competent in these areas before they were given responsibility for undertaking them in the clinical setting. At the same time, we perceived competency in any one of these areas as incorporating important elements of communication, understanding and reflection. In the case of aseptic technique (maintaining a sterile field), for example, it might be important to assess not only that the students' technique was correct but that they understood their reasons for carrying out the procedure, were aware of the possible effects on the patient of their actions and knew what complications to look for. In order to assess these factors it was necessary to encapsulate more than just the skill in the assessment criteria.

In the case of aseptic technique, we designed an assessment that was closely linked to laboratory sessions students had undertaken. The *Mrs Henderson* learning package focused on a young woman undergoing mastectomy for carcinoma of the breast. The laboratory session accompanying this package had the students dressing Mrs Henderson's mastectomy wound post-operatively. The aseptic technique assessment was derived from this package and required students to teach Mrs Henderson aseptic technique so that she could care for her wound once discharged. This was a realistic situation as Mrs Henderson had discharged herself three days post-operatively. Students were thus required to develop a teaching plan for Mrs Henderson and implement this in a role-play situation.

This assessment required students to do much more than simply repeat a formula for a procedure. They were required to understand thoroughly the principles and concepts underlying the procedure and to be able to communicate them clearly and appropriately to their client. Students were provided with assessment criteria in advance of the assessment and once these criteria were met students could perform this skill under supervision in the clinical setting. An example of assessment criteria given in advance is outlined in Chapter 8. Similar assessments frameworks were developed for credentialling of the other 'cornerstone' skills.

Facilitation in the laboratory

Facilitation in the laboratory varies from one session to the next, depending on the design. For sessions like the guided imagery laboratory only one facilitator per group (fifteen to twenty students) was required. It was important, however, that facilitators conducting this session were sufficiently skilled and comfortable doing so. For other sessions such as the peritoneal dialysis laboratory a ratio of one facilitator for every eight students was used; this ratio usually requires employment of additional staff. In our case we used clinical facilitators. The use of clinical facilitators enables them to be more successfully integrated into the teaching team and also emphasises consistency with what is practised on-campus and in the clinical setting. As is the case with problem-based tutorials, facilitator guides are provided if particular specialist knowledge is required by the facilitator. An example of the facilitator guide for the peritoneal dialysis laboratory is included in Appendix 6.

Facilitating in the laboratory can be very enjoyable and provides an informal environment for the exchange of ideas, knowledge, feelings and experiences. Students can be quite convivial, taking on both the role-play and activities with varying degrees of seriousness depending on the subject-matter. The laboratory has proved to be an environment in which very sensitive issues can be explored and at the same time one in which students can really enjoy the process of learning.

One of the first laboratory sessions students in the course encounter is an activities of daily living laboratory where they explore the intricacies of bed baths, shaving others, showering, washing a bed-ridden person's hair and so on. Students wear their swimming costumes and practise on each other. Initially they are quite incredulous at the thought that we are serious about the laboratory; in spite of their reservations, however, it is a laboratory that they always enjoy and learn from. As the recipients of their peers' nursing actions they provide excellent feedback to each other. They describe in detail just how comfortable or uncomfortable every action is and are full of helpful suggestions.

Evaluation of laboratories

Laboratory sessions have been evaluated alongside learning packages on the forms outlined in Appendix 8. Student comments regarding laboratories have tended to refer to the length of time provided to undertake activities, the amount of facilitator and equipment resources provided and whether the activities were helpful. Their suggestions have been taken into account when running the sessions again or in designing similar ones. There has also been a fair degree of informal evaluation when students feed back information during problem-based tutorials. This information is then relayed to those who designed the laboratory session during team meetings to ensure a thorough evaluation of the success of the laboratory for future reference.

Conclusion

In this chapter we have shown how laboratory sessions can be developed to complement the problem-based learning process. These sessions can be crafted to meet the individual student learning needs for any particular package. In the case of nursing, such sessions have enabled students to gauge more accurately how they will manage in their practice as nurses. This has been achieved by using the physical space of the laboratory and by carefully structuring the laboratory sheets and sessions to follow explicitly the process of clinical reasoning and decision-making. Such a framework can be easily adapted for any professional practice. We hope we have conveyed through these examples a sense of the enormous potential of laboratory learning.

Chapter 6
Integrating knowledges in clinical practice

Marie Cooke

Through problem-based learning I was able to identify SINIs with the clients I looked after. Group process taught me to get along with and participate in the health-care team. Self-directed learning allowed me to research during clinical if the need arose. And, communication was important for the client, in developing a rapport, and in the health-care team to obtain, share and use information.

Liz, student

In this chapter we illustrate the integration of clinical experiences within a problem-based nursing course. We consider the clinical issues arising from this approach; the factors involved in integrating on- and off-campus learning; and the development and differences of clinical experiences across the three years of the degree. Using information drawn from a survey, the chapter outlines student responses to the structure and implementation of clinical practice. (The survey is discussed more fully in Appendix 7.) Although the discussion in this chapter relates to clinical experiences within an undergraduate nursing degree, the design and processes outlined can be translated to any course that involves a practical component.

In putting together a practice-based generalist course the challenge is to structure the course to allow transfer and integration of learning from a number of knowledge areas. For nursing this means that the emphasis in the course structure is on promoting learning which can be transferred to and integrated with a number of clinical situations. One way to do this is by designing the learning around broad concept areas. Rather than basing part of a semester's work around content specific to a practice area of a discipline or profession, such as psychiatry or midwifery, a semester course can be made up of two or more modules with each module having a particular focus and core concepts. The core concepts and focus then direct the theme for the learning experiences both on- and off-campus.

For example, a focus for a module in a generalist nursing course may be Health, Culture and Care, with core concepts such as transcultural and indigenous nursing issues, health, wellness and culture. The learning materials might then consist of learning packages which situate the student as a school health nurse dealing with such typical adolescent issues as concerns about weight, skin or sexuality; might engage students in community and primary health issues; or might situate students in positions which require them to consider transcultural and indigenous issues. The clinical experiences integrated within this module might thus consist of such activities as students (i) interviewing adolescents about health-related issues, (ii) conducting small-scale community assessments, (iii) interviewing migrants about health-related issues or (iv) investigating community-based primary health-care facilities. Such a structure puts the emphasis on the generic practice of nursing and develops a more holistic approach to client care which will provide graduates with the knowledge and skills for beginning practice in all settings, and which requires students to integrate their knowledge of diverse elements such as community health policy and microbiology. It encourages students to conceptualise those aspects of nursing that are common to all settings in which nurses work (psychiatric, maternity, community, etc.) and all focuses (health and wellness and health breakdown) so that learning can be transferred to a variety of clinical situations.

Integrating clinical experiences

In the use of a concept-based structure as well as an approach which structures the learning around problems derived from professional practice, a number of challenges arise for designing and implementing clinical experiences. The clinical experiences must further encourage the characteristics embodied in this approach, for example, self-directive and active learning, integration of theory and practice, problem-solving and clinical reasoning skills. Clinical experiences must also focus on the modular core concepts in the clinical setting in which the student is placed. Since each on-campus learning package embodies specific concepts and specific learning, the clinical activities also need to incorporate specific knowledges. In order for the integrity and quality of the focus to be maintained, it is important that activities are structured as learning stimuli consistent with the problem-based nature of the course.

In our course, for example, students are placed in a variety of clinical settings during a module entitled Nursing and Adaptation. The core concepts of the module – stress, coping, self-esteem, control/choice, independence/dependence and activities of living – emanate from the overall theme of adaptation and its consequences for self-care. Thus, the clinical activities planned for students in relation to this module require them to focus on the core concepts in the clinical setting in which they are placed. The clinical placement associated with the module

Nursing and Adaptation is the first occasion students are placed in hospital and domiciliary nursing settings to learn. Examples of the activities students are required to undertake in their clinical placement are given in Figure 6.1. Because students are placed in a range of different settings – for example, community, medical, surgical, maternity and psychiatric – they will carry out the activities in their particular setting.

Activity 1: Learning goals

This activity requires you to identify your learning needs, goals and actions to assist you to develop self-directed learning strategies.

(i)   Identify 3 personal learning goals for this clinical experience and give to your clinical facilitator on Monday. You may wish to develop these goals utilising ward profiles and in consultation with the nursing staff in your allocated area.

(ii) Briefly describe in writing how you might go about meeting these goals, and give this to your clinical facilitator on Monday.

(iii) Reflect on one of these goals and discuss this at the debriefing session on Friday.

(iv) Evaluate, in writing, your strategies for achieving each of your goals in terms of their effectiveness, and hand to your clinical facilitator on Friday.

Activity 2

This activity focuses on some of the concepts you have visited in Nursing and Adaptation. Describe the sights and sounds you notice in your clinical placement setting.

What are the feelings associated with these sights and sounds? Describe them below.

How do you feel in the role of a nursing student? Can you imagine yourself as a registered nurse?

Focus on how you think you will *adapt* to this environment and to your role as a nursing student.

What resources are available to you?
Outline some strategies for promoting your own *self-care*.
Share your responses with your clinical group and/or your facilitator.

Activity 3

This activity allows you to integrate some of the nursing practices you have learnt in the clinical setting. With your clinical facilitator, organise to be involved in some elements of client care within the limits of your practice. These activities could include vital signs assessment and recording, and assistance with the activities of daily living. Before you become involved, think about how you feel about interacting (communicating and using nursing practice skills) with the client? What are the challenges/difficulties for you?

How might you deal with these?
What resources are available to you?

Figure 6.1:   Clinical learning activities

Preparatory and reflective activities – facilitators and students

The range of learning opportunities that arise during clinical practice is enormous, and these learning opportunities are difficult to simulate on-campus. This makes facilitation of student enquiry in the clinical environment crucial. Since full-time faculty need to be supported by casual registered nurses in order to maintain a safe ratio of facilitators to students during clinical practice, the role of part-time staff becomes an important issue. It is vital for the integrity of the course that clinical facilitators be fully aware of the nature and elements of problem-based learning, and of the characteristics of facilitation which may be different from their previous ideas about clinical teaching. Part-time clinical facilitators benefit greatly from support provided through orientation and support sessions. As the lynch-pin between helping students to fulfil the requirements of the course and supporting them in the achievement of their learning goals, clinical facilitators encounter many difficulties. Often it is the clinical facilitator who is required to negotiate with agency staff on behalf of the students and of the course for any number of matters including:

- explaining students' behaviours, for example, their questioning approach;
- reinforcing that students' university learning is legitimate;
- resisting agency staffs' attempts to use students as part of daily staffing numbers;
- removing students from the clinical area for impromptu tutorials.

To this end, clinical facilitators must have a commitment to the learning strategy used and it is vital that this is recognised and that explicit action is taken to assist clinical facilitators to adapt to their role. Problem-based orientation workshops must be held regularly for all clinical facilitators as they begin work. An important feature of such workshops is the opportunity for clinical facilitators to join a group of students working through learning material with the assistance of a full-time facilitator. Such an experience helps new clinical staff to understand both facilitation and the nature of the learning strategies, so that these may be continued off-campus. That is, the ways in which students' enquiry and clinical decision-making skills are encouraged need to be emphasised in order for these skills to be further promoted and developed in the clinical setting. Interestingly, students' comments after their first few clinical placements highlighted this aspect, suggesting that they engaged in client situations in a manner similar to the way in which they work through learning packages. Year 3 students' comments also verify the relationship between on- and off-campus learning.

I would describe problem-based learning as holistic primary nursing – focusing on clients' situations and incorporating all facets of nursing in one – This has an advantage because when you are on clinical it is easy to relate to a real client and the problems that can occur with complex health breakdown.

Erica, Year 3 student

Throughout each semester pre-clinical conferences and debriefing sessions are held for both clinical facilitators and students, as means by which expectations, learning needs, assessment and other issues may be discussed and clarified. During evaluation of the course students have identified that careful preparation makes their clinical experience more rewarding and useful. Students encounter many situations which they say cause them some degree of anxiety. Typical are:

- trying any new task is always a bit worrying for the first time;
- never worked or cared for men before; felt embarrassed at having to see them naked and shower or bathe them;
- not sure of what I could say about the patient's condition or how to answer patient's questions;
- staff attitudes towards university nursing students;
- dealing with people who were dying;
- dealing with the mentally ill;
- crisis situations eg. patient emergencies, fires, etc.

It is important to acknowledge these concerns and provide opportunities for students to prepare for clinical experiences both on- and off-campus.

Debriefing sessions are especially important for both facilitators and students. Facilitator debriefing sessions consider what has worked well and what has not worked well. Often, the issues which are identified as not having worked well can be used as trigger material for facilitators to process. This has been found to be an effective strategy since it is similar to the ways in which students engage with learning material. As well as modelling the enquiry process used in problem-based learning, it assists facilitators to identify ways in which changes can be made at either the individual level or the course-structure level. Another strategy used to involve part-time clinical facilitators with the problem-based course is to encourage their participation in on-campus skill development laboratories and on-campus skills assessments and in fixed-resource sessions.

Although clinical facilitators usually provide a debriefing session for students throughout clinical practice placements as required, it is useful to hold further debriefing sessions on-campus throughout the course. Such sessions have been conducted as small-group meetings where students reflect and share clinical experiences which they found difficult, rewarding or challenging. Difficult

1. In your group spend some time identifying your experiences of Registered Nurses.

2. In pairs, outline some of the interpersonal skills you have identified as being important for you to develop further as you move towards becoming registered nurses.

   What resources are available to help you?

   What might hinder you?

   What sorts of principles might guide you?

3. We'll spend some time simulating responses to the following scenarios and identifying strategies to deal with them effectively.

(a) You are newly registered and working in the emergency department. It is your second day. The charge nurse asks you to assess a 2-year-old girl in a cubicle with her mother. You carry out observations and ask the child's mother what seems to be the problem. She tells you that her daughter has been sexually assaulted.

   How do you respond:
   – to the mother?
   – to the charge nurse?
   – to the child?

   How do you feel?

(b) Tom Sanders is admitted having taken an overdose of 'sleeping tablets' some time earlier. He is drowsy. You spend some time with Tom after his gastric lavage, talking about some of the reasons for his despair. The charge nurse calls you out and, although the department is quiet, she tells you not to waste your time.

   How might you respond?

   How do you feel?

(c) Emma Gray is an 80-year-old lady who was admitted several hours ago from a nursing home. You have not been caring for her but as you walk past her cubicle you see that she looks uncomfortable and that her mouth is so dry that she can't swallow.

   What is your response?

(d) You are met on your first day by the Registered Nurse who says 'you're one of those university-trained nurses, I suppose I'll have to spoon-feed you'.

   How might you respond?

   How do you feel?

(e) Fred Smith is a 52-year-old man who came into the A&E to have an infected sore on his right hand attended to. He is homeless and lives with several other men under the Grey Street Bridge. The treatment of his hand has been completed and the charge nurse tells you to show Fred to the door; she wants you not to get 'sentimental' about him as 'these people' are all alike. As Fred gathers up his (meagre) belongings you notice that he is without shoes, and outside it is a cold, wet night.

Figure 6.2:   Debriefing activity sheet

experiences have often resulted from interactions with agency staff where the values embodied in the course have been questioned or commented upon negatively. For example, some agency staff commented that students 'are too questioning', although such questioning is a deliberate educational policy. In order to make sure that they are fully informed about what students are capable of and the approach they take, nursing staff at the agencies at which students are placed also require regular workshops/information sessions about the nature and structure of the course. An example of activities which have been used to assist students during debriefing sessions is given in Figure 6.2. The scenarios used were some situations related to teaching staff by students from their previous clinical experiences.

The promotion of enquiry, processing, clinical decision-making and self-direction skills continues throughout the three years of the degree. As the course progresses the clinical activities demand a greater ability to integrate a number of complex concepts as well as to promote more self-direction. By Year 3 the students generally require little facilitation in the clinical environment. This is sometimes a problem for agency staff but the students feel pleased about being able to be fairly autonomous.

Figure 6.3 gives an example of an activity for Year 3 students.

Activity 1

In consultation with your facilitator draw up a learning contract which:

1. Identifies your learning goals and time-frames for achieving these in the 6-week clinical experience. (You may need to take into account your own needs; needs identified by the clinical agency; needs which allow you to complete your self-directed community experience and the nature of the clinical placement area.)

2. Outlines the information you need to gather in order to meet your identified learning goals. (This information might come from literature, resource persons, policy documents, ward profiles, etc.)

3. Identifies the activities/interactions which may facilitate the achievement of these goals.

4. Develops criteria to evaluate the extent to which you meet your learning goals.

5. Identifies the people you consider would be able to evaluate appropriately the achievement of identified goals and from whom you could obtain feedback.

Steps 1–5 need to be completed 3 weeks before your clinical placement to allow time for this to be communicated to agencies and facilitators/preceptors.

On return to the university write an account which analyses the extent to which you were able to meet your learning goals; the effectiveness of your criteria; and any factors which helped or hindered your ability to achieve the identified learning goals. Include the evaluation undertaken during your clinical experience using the criteria you developed.

Figure 6.3:   Year 3 activity

The sort of feedback that comes from agencies in response to the question 'what has worked well' tends to be of this kind:

- well-defined goals, strategies and evaluation criteria;
- students have taken advantage of learning opportunities in the ward;
- pre-reading prior to the students' arrival and gaining an insight into the aim of their work experience;
- worked with enthusiasm, showed initiative, keen to learn and be involved.

In encouraging an increasing level of self-direction during the degree, preceptorship for Year 3 students is an exciting and real opportunity for students to expand their knowledge, skills and attitudes safely by working continuously with a staff member from the agency. ('Preceptorships emerged in the early 1960s to assist students in their transition from student to graduate nurse. Preceptors are members of a clinical nursing staff who work with students and new graduates on a one-to-one basis to provide guidance and supervision in the clinical area' (Zerbe and Lachat 1991:18).) It allows students to gain immediate feedback on performance and makes it easier for them to make the transition to the professional role. Two Year 3 students' responses to the question 'What aspects of problem-based learning were useful in the clinical setting?' outline what they see as helping them make the transition to clinical practice:

- problem-framing; the ability to apply clinical reasoning skills; the support obtained from peers and facilitators; assertion skills supported goal attainment; reflection promoted personal and professional growth, and learning; teamwork–communication
- lab sessions; self-directed research and study; group process; communication skills

Students' perceptions of clinical experiences

Future development of the clinical experiences integrated within the problem-based nursing degree have required evaluation of the overall nature of these experiences and related issues. To this end, a study was undertaken of Year 1 students' perceptions of facilitation characteristics and certain aspects of the problem-based course pre- and post-clinical. This gave insight into the implementation and structure of clinical experiences and is shown in Appendix 7. Students' responses to the pre- and post-clinical surveys provide useful information for staff development, restructuring of nursing laboratories and assessment within the degree. A similar study has been undertaken with second and third year students in order to investigate what might be the similarities and differences for these students.

The survey indicates that students value the support provided by a facilitator who is cognizant of the philosophy of problem-based learning, which places the student at the centre of the learning and values students' contributions to the learning process. This is further borne out by students' responses regarding facilitator assistance during clinical experiences. Although facilitator assistance included supportive, preparatory, instructive and evaluative behaviours, supportive behaviours were most commonly mentioned by students. Examples of comments on these behaviours include:

- reassurance – talking about what happened;
- university facilitator excellent in assisting all of us to work through our problems and encouraging us to express ourselves;
- encouragement and support;
- encouraged me to talk about situation and feelings I had;
- talked us through the experience and discussed our reactions, implications for nursing and future experiences.

Of all the characteristics, 'Encourages student initiative' was found to be more effective post-clinically than was anticipated in the pre-clinical survey. This finding suggests that facilitators were able to create an environment where students were able to have more control over their learning and behaviour in clinical situations so that they could achieve the aims of independent thought and initiative. This is not always the case, as Blainey suggests:

> many of us have given students a difficult double message. We have said, 'Be independent; be risk takers; be change agents; be self-directed in your learning; never make a mistake; there is no room for errors in nursing.' We can reduce anxiety and increase learning by creating a climate for learning in which less-than-perfect-behaviour at new skills and application of knowledge is acceptable.
>
> (Blainey 1980:35)

'Provides feedback through evaluation' was experienced by students as very effective. Other studies have shown that students identified evaluation/assessment as anxiety-producing in clinical situations (Sellek 1982; Kleehammer *et al.* 1990; Jones 1978), whereas the present inquiry suggests that students find the evaluative role valuable in dealing with difficult/challenging situations. These contrasting results may reflect the actual role of the clinical facilitator in a different learning environment. As well, the philosophy, structure and implementation of assessment within the course may have been reflected in how useful students perceived the 'evaluative' role of clinical facilitators to be; this will be more fully detailed in Chapter 8 on assessment within the problem-based course.

Of all the population groups, students aged 31–50 generally rated (post-clinical) facilitation characteristics lower than all other groups, especially 'Acknowledges student priorities', 'Clarifies learning contracts' and 'Provides feedback through evaluation'. As the majority of these students indicated that they had had previous experience, it would be expected that the characteristics listed above might assist them with their particular learning needs. It may be that their experience was a hindrance because facilitators may have given priority to inexperienced students, or these mature students may have used their personal resources in dealing with clinical situations. These issues need to be considered when developing practical experiences in any discipline area. Although students are encouraged to develop their own learning goals for each placement, the other activities designed to trigger learning need to be flexible enough to allow students with different needs to identify and achieve their individual learning requirements as well as achieve their identified goals.

The eleven facilitation characteristics adapted from the Bachelor of Nursing submission document (Griffith University 1990) were, on the whole, ranked by students as effective. This information is useful in supporting the aims of clinical facilitation and, as such, may help clarify the role for facilitators. Clinical facilitators who are new to the course find the role confusing as the student is usually 'buddied' with a registered nurse and spends most of the clinical time with this person. Facilitation and the role of facilitators both on- and off-campus has been further discussed in Chapter 3.

As well as responding to characteristics of clinical facilitation, students were asked to document their perceptions of nine aspects of the course. The information gained from student responses provided valuable information for staff development and course evaluation. Experienced students found that 'Working through laboratory sheets for skill development' was least useful. This possibly reflects some sense of frustration with having to work through skill sheets for skills that they may have been practising for some time as assistants-in-nursing or enrolled nurses. In fact, this was confirmed by one experienced student who ranked this aspect quite low post-clinically but wrote 'not because they weren't useful but I'm already competent at the skills'.

Before starting their clinical experience most Year 1 students perceived 'Being responsible for your own learning' as not very useful. Although this is a major goal of the problem-based focus, it is not surprising that students perceived this to have a low priority because, at the beginning of Year 1, some students are unused to and resent having to take responsibility for their own learning. The nurturing of self-directed learners is a difficult task, requiring considerable skill from the facilitator.

As Brookfield (1986:11) suggests, students are all at differing levels of ability for self-direction. From my own and others' experience (Brookfield 1986; Little and Ryan 1988), some students seem to flourish in this environment, some are intimidated by the process, some resist and yet others become quite angry. The major issue evident here is that most students find the process so different from their previous experiences with education that initially they are unable to understand and appreciate its significance or its liberating potential.

The change when students finished their clinical experience for Year 1 was dramatic: 'Being responsible for your own learning' was now found to be one of the most useful of the aspects. This finding reflects a growing acceptance of self-direction and the opportunities and benefits it holds. This was certainly borne out by one student who chose to rank this as very useful and wrote beside it 'but it took me till Semester 2 to realise this'. It is also evident from the Year 3 student responses to their last clinical placement that they valued their self-directedness and believed they had acquired valuable skills, through the problem-based learning process, which allowed them to learn and gain access to information in any situation.

All students found 'Being able to have certain skills credentialled (assessed) on-campus' one of the most useful aspects of the course. Situations which involve students performing, or not performing, psychomotor skills do concern students, as the following student responses regarding difficult clinical situations indicate:

- first injections
- giving medication
- using practical skills on patients
- saying no to giving drugs (I had not been assessed).

The reasons students gave for finding psychomotor skills difficult referred to feeling nervous or insecure, not feeling confident and the risks involved for the client. It would seem then that the process by which student have skills assessed on-campus (see Chapters 5 and 8 for a description of this process) may help to overcome some of the difficulties experienced during clinical experience. It is, however, important to teach and assess psychomotor skills by highlighting their importance in relation to the client's whole situation, rather than teaching them as a series of steps to be achieved. As was outlined in the preceding chapter, it is also important to allow students to deal with their feelings about certain issues within the nursing laboratory either before or after clinical placements.

It is evident from the following responses that it is not always the skill *per se* which concerns students, but rather a composite of doing something and the emotions involved:

- coming to terms with nudity of other sex when showering them;
- it was bathing old women – it just felt odd and I didn't know how they would react;
- unsure how to handle the male genital area without causing embarrassment to patient and me.

It is important, then, that clinical facilitators assist students with the difficulties they encounter in the clinical environment. Students have indicated that this assistance is often achieved by supporting them, sometimes by offering guidance. Typical facilitator behaviours that students appreciated were identified as follows:

- by rehearsing the procedure and being available to give assistance;
- encouraging confidence with procedure;
- reassuring – talking about what happened;
- by introducing me to the client chosen and opening an informal talk with the client;
- acting as a sounding board;
- facilitator talked it through and helped me identify ways of approaching situation.

The findings obtained from evaluation of aspects of the course and of effective facilitation characteristics are valuable in terms of the on-going development and planning of the course. The former provide information for re-working the course, and the latter (the perceived and experienced effectiveness of the facilitation characteristics) will be useful information in the on-going design and implementation of staff development courses for clinical facilitators.

Conclusion

The discussion in this chapter has illustrated the challenges and issues associated with integrating practical experiences within a problem-based learning course. It has considered the importance of maintaining and furthering the processes inherent in the learning strategy in the clinical environment. Examples of clinical activities have been provided to illustrate the consistency of the clinical learning stimuli with those used on-campus and the increasing self-directedness of the students. Year 1 and Year 3 students' responses to clinical experiences highlight the advantages of the learning strategy as it integrates theory and practice, encouraging problem-solving, clinical reasoning and communication and teamwork skills.

Chapter 7
Helping teachers to help students learn

Christine Alavi

Throughout this book we have tried to convey our enthusiasm for problem-based learning. It must be said, however, that such a way of learning poses its own difficulties, for both students and staff. For the teacher what seems appealing in this way of helping students to learn can involve a difficult transition from a more traditional teaching role, and this is sometimes a bar to the implementation of a problem-based course. There must be open acknowledgement of these difficulties, and this chapter attempts to give some suggestions about how to help teachers make a successful transition from teacher to facilitator. We will draw on our own experience to show how staff can be helped to understand and feel more comfortable with the facilitative role. We will discuss staff orientation; ways of organising sessions for helping staff to continue to develop skills in problem-based learning; and staff selection. Here, and in practice, we insist on the importance of continuing reflection on, and sharing of, facilitation experiences.

Most teachers have been prepared through courses in which acculturation as a teacher, while it may include problem-solving and experiential elements, concentrates on the role of imparting information and developing the curriculum as an individual expert within a particular subject area. When people come to work in a problem-based course they are often confronted with questions about what their role is, the role of students, and a variety of expectations of the course. While the different approach of problem-based learning can seem exciting and challenging, it can often lead to anxiety and to a feeling of being deskilled. This in turn can lead to a retreat into defensiveness and a wish to give lectures and return to more conventional tutorial sessions – in other words, to regain teacher control. Facilitators may feel even more discomfited by the students' initial desire for the teacher to be a purveyor of information, someone who gives answers and does not expect them to take the major responsibility for their own learning.

At such times there is a need for staff to hold on to a fundamental belief in the process – particularly when questions such as 'Is it going to work?' circulate in the student body, and in your own mind. In order to overcome these feelings of insecurity, and maintain a problem-based focus, it is important for new staff to be thoroughly orientated to the course, and for all staff to continue to reflect on their practice as facilitators. In our view such sessions are the single most important contribution to the success of a problem-based course.

Orientation

For people coming into an existing course, the most effective orientation strategies are those which allow new academics the opportunity for practical experience with time for reflection on those experiences – strategies which mirror the processes which students undergo. Since, by its very nature, a problem-based course involves continuous evaluation, it is essential from the outset that peer support and evaluation, self-evaluation and student evaluation are seen as being valued and carried out as a matter of course, as well as not being experienced as threatening. An atmosphere like this can be created from the new staff member's initial introduction to a problem-based course, and a deliberate and responsive orientation can help to minimise fears.

It is sometimes difficult to know where to start when developing orientation sessions because of the desire to give background information in order to contextualise the problem-based process, as well as to give some meaningful 'hands-on' experience as a facilitator. One way of combining both these needs most effectively is to present the orientation sessions so that they resemble a typical learning package like the ones students experience. In presenting the sessions this way staff are able to work co-operatively to identify situations in need of improvement for themselves, and to explore some of the ways in which to seek the information needed to resolve those situations.

Strategies that we have found useful have included the deliberate creation of a climate of acceptance; some active exposure to problem-based learning; sharing of experiences by both staff and students; role-modelling of the facilitative process; an introduction to the development of trigger material and learning packages; and an opportunity for reflection for those already initiated, who have some experience of working in a problem-based course. These are all vital elements and can easily be overlooked if their importance is not consistently underlined and if there is insufficient time to reflect on, and make explicit, what is happening in the orientation course.

We have used varying approaches to orientation sessions, and the timetable shown in Figure 7.1 is a hybrid course developed as a result of our experiences in planning orientation sessions over the first three years of our course.

Such a course introduces new staff to problem-based learning but is merely the beginning of on-going activities to develop and deepen understanding of the

Day 1	Introductions. A display of students' work across the years. Creating a climate of acceptance.
	Block material to trigger issues of facilitation in problem-based learning–working in a group.
	Feedback from group processing – leading to questions for the fixed resource sessions for the next day.
	Reflection on the day's activities.
Day 2	Fixed resource sessions dealing with university issues, and facilitation in problem-based learning.
	Group-building exercises.
	Introduction to the development of learning packages.
	Reflection on the day's activities.
Day 3	Small groups with one member practising as facilitator, each facilitator using learning packages from the year in which they themselves will be working.
	Debrief on this activity – whole group.
	Reflection on the day.
Day 4	Work with students in a group, processing a learning package.
	Facilitated by an experienced facilitator. Perhaps co-facilitating.
	Reflection on the day.
Day 5	Meet in teaching teams to discuss themes and plans.
	Reflection on the week. Plans for ongoing support and education sessions.

Figure 7.1:   An orientation course

processes which form the basis of problem-based learning. A detailed description of the activities outlined in Figure 7.1 follows to give you a clearer sense of what is involved.

Day 1

A display of students' work across the years
New staff are often amazed, as we are, at the creativity and diversity of students' collaborative and individual work. Sometimes staff teaching across different years have little idea of the work which has been done in other years. A display of students' work, which will typically include videos, posters, models, educational pamphlets and photographs; is a useful way of seeing what students achieve, as well as giving ideas for activities outside the usual range.

Creating a climate of acceptance

In fostering a climate of acceptance, it is important not only to create a welcoming atmosphere, but to have available for the new staff members all the documentation related to the course so that they may read it at their leisure and ask questions as they arise. It is ideal if all new staff can join the faculty at the same time, preferably some weeks before the students begin classes, so that a cohesive group can be formed which acknowledges and uses the experience and expertise of all members. Introductions, acknowledgements of what each person is bringing to the course, as well as the sharing of ideas about problem-based learning, can stimulate discussion and give staff members some initial knowledge about each other.

Block material to trigger facilitation issues

If staff work through a block of learning material they are able to have some hands-on experience from the very first day. New staff working through such material will have a similar experience to that of students carrying out the same activity. Rather than identifying situations in need of improvement for the client in the block material, however, they are encouraged to identify situations in need of improvement for themselves as they facilitate such a learning package. Figure 7.2 introduces the activity.

You are facilitating the block of learning material below with a group of first-year students. Read through the material and identify what are the situations in need of improvement for you as the facilitator:

You are a registered nurse working in the psychiatric unit at Nathan Hospital. You have been asked to go to the emergency department to see a new patient, Greg Stone.

Mr Stone is in a cubicle with his father. He is scruffy, dirty, and rather malodorous. He is gazing through a circle formed by his thumb and index finger, and occasionally claps his hands and shakes his wrists violently.

You say hello to Mr Stone and he responds with 'The answers are blowing in the wind.' Then he tells you that he is Jim Morrison and that he played in a band with Lou Reed.

You find it difficult to decipher what Mr Stone is saying to you because for much of the time he seems to be speaking gibberish. You ask his father how long Greg has been behaving in this way. He tells you that he has been behaving 'strangely' for 5 or 6 days, and that earlier today he walked into a stranger's house with his motorcycle helmet on chanting and 'talking nonsense'.

Figure 7.2:   A block to trigger facilitation issues

Facilitators usually identify that they believe this material is too difficult for first-year students; that they feel unable to facilitate it because it falls outside their area of knowledge; or, perhaps, that such material has little place in a generalist nursing course.

They are then encouraged to work through the block of material very much as we asked you to do in Chapter 1. They find that they do have a good deal of prior knowledge, that many of the situations in need of improvement which they identify for Greg Stone are generalisable. They also have the opportunity to see an expert facilitator work through this material with them, and to reflect on the experience once the activity is over. They are also encouraged to generate questions arising from the material, or from facilitation, which can be addressed in the fixed resource session the following day.

Reflection on this day might evaluate the usefulness of the process framework, allowing participants the opportunity to share their understandings about the material presented so far.

Day 2

Fixed resource sessions

Usually the first hour of the second day is taken up with questions stimulated by the activities of day 1. Questions can be answered and further discussion can be stimulated.

Group-building exercises

Figure 7.3 shows a group-building exercise which can be conducted by someone outside the school; usually a behavioural scientist is the most appropriate person to do this.

Introduction to developing learning packages

Learning packages are the structure on which the process of problem-based learning hangs. The methods of developing such packages have been described and discussed in Chapter 2, but it is important to say here that, if new staff are not introduced – with their knowledge being developed during future sessions – to how and why learning packages are developed, it is very difficult for them to grasp the 'big picture' of a problem-based learning course. An introduction could provide exposure to the raw clinical data with examples of how this has been formed into learning packages, offering them the opportunity to ask questions and explaining that workshops which deal with how to do this will be a vital part of further development sessions. Such an introduction is probably as much as can be coped with at this time in a one-week orientation package. However, if you

Our overall aim is to develop the foundations for an effective and supportive teaching team. We will be attempting to achieve this by working through the following:

Past focus	(aim: to surface and tidy up any relevant 'unfinished business' or loose ends)
	What attracted you to apply for your job?
	What did you feel about the selection and hiring process (eg. any hitches, delays, inconveniences, resentments, etc.)?
	How do you feel about being here in the school right now (eg. impressions, atmosphere, etc.)?
Sharing of ideas	Summarise themes
Present focus	(aim: to reflect on the present course facing the team)
	What interests or excites you about the course?
	What initial concerns or anxieties, if any, do you have about the course, your role, yourself in the course?
Team sharing	Summarise group themes
Future focus	(aim: to decide on the kind of working relationship you wish to create together to enhance your course effectiveness)
	What do the excitements and concerns expressed by team members indicate in concrete terms, for your development as an effective and supportive working team?
Team sharing	What ongoing mechanisms for monitoring, evaluating and learning from our team do we need to put in place?

Figure 7.3:   Group-building exercises
Source: Keithia Wilson 1991

are fortunate enough to have a longer time period available then the development of learning packages could comprise a much larger part of the orientation period.

Reflection on day 2 may extend the group process, and will allow further exploration and discussion about the development of learning packages.

Day 3

Small group activities
Such activities can typically involve groups of four or five staff members working together with one of them acting as the facilitator while the others work through

a block of material from a learning package which students will use. These activities have the advantages that facilitation skills can be practised in a safe environment with feedback from other members of the group; that another perspective on the problem-based process can be gained; and that some familiarity is gained with the sorts of learning packages which have already been developed. Full group discussion and reflection following this activity will enable a more comprehensive discussion on facilitation, with staff members sharing strategies and learning from each other.

Day 4

Working with students

Another strategy which might be helpful is for an experienced facilitator to work through a block of learning material with students who have volunteered to come to the university for this purpose. Such a demonstration may be carried out live or may already have been video-taped. The advantages of the former are that new staff can join the student group and experience the process firsthand, while the advantages of the latter are that the video-tape can be stopped at any stage for questions. In either case new staff members have the opportunity to see the facilitative role modelled, and to ask questions about particular strategies. New staff might also co-facilitate such a session and gain feedback from the experienced facilitator as well as from students in the group.

For off-campus clinical facilitators and for those who might find difficulty attending orientation sessions, a self-directed package such as the one we introduced you to in Chapter 1 has proved valuable orientation to problem-based learning. This can be augmented by a video-tape which shows typical situations that students might encounter in the clinical setting and how these can be facilitated. Such a package can be followed up by telephone or personal contact to address specific concerns or questions. By day 4 there is likely to be a more relaxed period of reflection at the end of the day. It can be valuable to summarise themes which can contribute to ongoing staff education sessions.

Day 5

Meeting in teaching teams

The focus of teaching will have been set before most new staff join the team. It is useful if some planning can be left until new people join the staff so that they feel some sense of ownership of the course. This meeting can be an introduction to the work of the year or semester in which the new staff member will work, and will involve some discussion of the focus, assessment, associated clinical activities and planning for future consultation.

Reflection

At all times during this orientation week, and throughout a problem-based course, the importance of reflection cannot be overstressed. It is particularly important in the orientation week not only to carry out the orientation activities, but also to make those activities explicit by reflecting on them at the end of each day, and then again in the last session of the week. It is imperative that reflection sessions be seen and accepted as a regular and integral part of the problem-based course.

On-going activities

Although orientation sessions are essential they provide only an introduction to problem-based learning. Regular sessions which extend and deepen the understanding and experience of facilitation within such a course, as well as extending its boundaries and repertoire, are vital. Although teaching and research commitments are heavy, most staff welcome these sessions as they give an opportunity for specific needs to be addressed. These sessions allow celebration of achievements and give an opportunity for staff to learn from each other. They also contribute to maintaining the integrity of the course by continual reflection.

Role-modelling the facilitative process

Some ways of modelling facilitation have already been outlined, and seeing facilitation demonstrated expertly is an excellent introduction. Other strategies which can be used as new facilitators become more comfortable in the role include having colleagues sit in and take part in tutorials and comment on facilitation strategies; taking time to observe others in the teaching team as they conduct tutorials; or video-taping facilitation and reviewing it later. On day 3 of the orientation we give new facilitators the opportunity to facilitate a small group of their peers as they work through a learning package. This gives a safe environment in which to take some first steps at facilitation. New facilitators have sometimes asked for these sessions to be video-taped so that they can compare their early performance as a facilitator with their developing performance.

The development of trigger materials

Further experience in the development of learning materials can be achieved by having new staff members work on an incomplete block of learning materials with a more experienced member, and take part in the evaluation of that learning package once it has been used by the students. This, in turn, leads to a deeper understanding of the role of assessment and evaluation in the course, as well as to the mechanics of how material is gathered and where it fits into the concept matrix for the course.

Another way of helping to develop skills in producing learning packages is to have members of the existing teaching team produce a video and identify the concepts to be drawn from it. The video could include such scenarios as a day in the life of a disabled person, an interaction in the classroom or an admission interview. New facilitators could view the video and identify triggers to address the concepts. The triggers could be written up as block material, or the video itself could be used as block material for which facilitators might produce a facilitators' guide.

Orientation in a new problem-based course

As was the case with the course we have been involved with, sometimes there is the challenge and opportunity to develop a course from the beginning. Although this may initially seem a daunting task, it can be achieved and we hope our experiences as described in this book will be helpful to those who might be about to embark on such development.

When we were given the task of developing a problem-based course there were a number of people who were able to help us. There was the Centre for the Advancement of Learning and Teaching within the university which had been involved in early planning about the course, and which had expertise in curriculum development in all its forms. This group was, however, unable to help with the specifics of a nursing course, and we were helped immeasurably by people at the School of Nursing at the University of Western Sydney who had a partially problem-based course. *Our* orientation consisted of visits to them to experience the day-to-day processes, and the orientation we have described in this book will, we hope, go some way to giving you a similar experience.

Support sessions

Support sessions may also have been identified at orientation as a need. Sometimes small *ad hoc* groups arise in response to specific facilitator concerns. For example, a common concern is that a facilitator is experiencing some difficulty in helping a student group sort out group process issues. Other facilitators might offer suggestions or reassurance, or may offer to sit in with the group to help to diagnose the problem. Such activities help further to develop confidence and trust between facilitators as well as increasing the range of facilitation strategies.

As well as supportive sessions which might address the philosophical and educational bases of problem-based learning, it is helpful if meetings which deal with more pragmatic and day-to-day issues are held regularly so that teaching teams can share understandings and clarify approaches to assessment, specific learning packages, course development and evaluation.

Staff selection

The way in which staff are selected to teach in a problem-based course is a major determinant of the ongoing success of the course. Potential employees must be provided with the information they need to make an informed decision about whether they wish to teach in such a course. Consistent with a problem-based learning approach, it is important that applicants be given opportunity to assimilate this information by having time to talk informally with the teaching team, and with students, and by attending problem-based tutorials and fixed-resource sessions. Supplying this information to applicants so that they have a better basis for their decision is as important as obtaining information about applicants. As well as the process of selection, the timing of appointments is important.

Staff should be appointed with sufficient time for them to take part in a thorough orientation course so that they can question their new role, practise in it and raise questions or concerns. This is particularly important for part-time and clinical staff, since not only will these people have less direct access to peer support and evaluation, but the integrity of the problem-based curriculum will be maintained only to the extent to which such staff feel integral to the course. Such time is well-spent because, if new staff do not have the opportunity for a thorough orientation, then there is more likelihood that difficulties will arise.

Conclusion

This chapter has discussed the ideals of staff orientation, and, while acknowledging that the ideal can not always be achieved, we would nevertheless want to stress the importance of incorporating regular reflection on what we do as teachers in a problem-based course. We would want to reiterate that effective and regular staff support and reflection are essential in fostering the on-going development of a problem-based course.

Chapter 8
Assessing problem-based learning

Christine Alavi and Marie Cooke

> *Supportive – I mean because it's non-competitive, we're not all out to get each other so if somebody has a problem you help them through it.*
>
> *Irene, student*

The ways in which assessment is structured in any course will have a major effect on how students learn. Assessment can be helpful for students' learning when it is integral to it, or it can merely concentrate on factual recall as is done in closed-book examinations, enticing students into rote learning. This chapter will discuss the processes and forms of assessment used within a problem-based course, showing how assessment criteria published in advance, integrated assessment items and teacher feedback enrich learning. It will also explain the role of group and individual assessment, giving examples derived from our experience. The chapter incorporates comments made by third-year students about their experiences of assessment.

Because assessment is an indication of what they will be rewarded for doing, assessment items must convince students in a problem-based learning course that self-direction, co-operative learning, collaboration and reflection are valued. If we say that we are wanting students to develop the ability to assess themselves and their peers, this too needs to be a component of assessment. If we state that students' learning is as important as what is learned, then we need to show students that we are not merely interested in the end products, but that the ways in which learning takes place will contribute to the grade they are given in any assessment item. Such learning 'how to learn' begins a life-long process by means of which students can continue to build on the learning that takes place in the course.

Integration of assessment

An important aim of the course is to help students integrate different areas of knowledge. When the teaching team is deciding on assessment items within a particular module, it devises an item which encourages students to bring together concepts from nursing, the sciences and the humanities in addressing some aspect

Describe a clinical situation you have experienced which relates to the concept of 'the good death'. Discuss and analyse this concept using the chosen situation, and integrate related concepts from nursing, humanities and the sciences, paying particular attention to such factors as quality of life, activities of living, crisis, bereavement, ethics, teamwork and co-ordination of care. What are the implications of your understanding of 'the good death' for your nursing practice in the chosen situation? Consider this from the client and her/his family and significant others' perspectives, and from your own perspective.

Figure 8.1: 'The good death'

of the module and its associated clinical experience. Sometimes the assessment items can be directly derived from the course material; it is always closely related to the Module. As an example, a Year 3 assessment item relating to a learning package dealing with palliative care is shown in Figure 8.1.

This assessment item incorporates both practical and theoretical elements, and integrates knowledges from various disciplines, in asking students to address concepts from Year 3 as they analyse a commonly occurring situation. The clinical experience associated with this item sees students undertaking experience in a hospice/palliative care unit.

Assessment criteria published in advance

In order for students to be able to prepare for assignments, and to help them identify how to satisfy the requirements of the assessment, the criteria by which assessments will be marked are published at the beginning of the semester. We publish criteria under four categories: Application of Theories and Concepts; Use of a Range of Formal and Informal Resources; Communication Skills; Contribution to Group Learning. These four categories are consistent across all years of the course. For the individual assessment item in Figure 8.1, the criteria and the categories are shown in Figure 8.2.

Feedback to students

In order for students to see assessment as integral to their learning it is valuable for teachers to give them regular and meaningful comments on their work. When the assessment item is marked, students are judged to have met the criteria at a 'well developed', 'developing' or 'unmet' level rather than being given a grade. The achievements that constitute these levels are determined by the teaching team as they develop the assessment item. The levels are explained to students and

1. *Application of Theories and Concepts*
   a. Clearly describes the circumstances of the chosen clinical situation.
   b. Demonstrates an understanding of the concept 'the good death'.
   c. Analyses the situation integrating concepts from nursing, humanities and the sciences (biological and behavioural) which address quality of life, activities of living, crisis, bereavement, ethics, teamwork and co-ordination of care.

2. *Use of a Variety of Formal and Informal Resources*
   Uses and integrates a range of formal and informal resources which reflect the concepts identified in 1c.

3. *Communication Skills*
   Presents the material in an appropriate academic format paying particular attention to consistent referencing, spelling and grammatical construction.

4. *Contribution to Group Learning*
   Provides a short discussion (500 words) reflecting on the extent to which you have obtained, shared and used information with members of your group.

Figure 8.2:   Categories and criteria for the 'good death' assignment

supported by extensive written feedback from the facilitator. A student who can apply concepts and theories, can use resources appropriately and can work co-operatively in a group may nevertheless have verbal or written communication difficulties. Such students will be provided with detailed facilitator comments to allow them to improve this area of their work. Should students receive an 'unmet' for any category, they have the opportunity to re-submit that assessment item. If categories continue to be unmet after a re-submission then the student will fail that assessment item, and may be offered a supplementary assessment, after the assessment board has considered their overall achievement. This supplementary assessment addresses concepts and skills similar to those in the original item.

Student 1

Application of Theories and Concepts (well developed)

Helen – you have described the clinical situation sensitively and with great detail and clarity. You have demonstrated that you have an in-depth understanding of 'the good death' for your client and her family. You have analysed and applied concepts from other disciplines and have integrated these appropriately. You have also identified how your own values and beliefs both helped and hindered your nursing care of the client, and have described the strategies you used to be more effective and to help you deal with your own grief.

Use of a Variety of Formal and Informal Resources (well developed)

There is evidence of wide reading and of extensive discussion with experts which you have integrated well into your assessment. You have used the resources to make comparisons which further your argument.

Communication Skills (developing)

You have written this well, with minimal spelling and grammatical errors. The assignment is well composed with a logical flow. Your referencing is inconsistent at times – please see pp. 4, 15 and 19 specifically.

Contribution to Group Learning (well developed)

Helen – you have obviously worked closely with other group members and have shared your resources. Your descriptions of this, and your reflections on it identify effective group process.

Student 2

Application of Theories and Concepts (unmet)

Margaret – although you have described the clinical situation many concepts are not explored in sufficient depth to demonstrate an understanding of 'the good death' for your client. Specifically your work would have been improved if you had analysed some of the ethical issues for yourself as they affected your ability to care for this client. You did not discuss the importance of teamwork except very cursorily, and so did not identify the supports available both to your client and yourself.

Use of a Variety of Formal and Informal Resources (developing)

There is evidence of the adequate use of formal resources but you have not really integrated these with your client situation. You do not discuss the positive and negative aspects of the resources you have used, but rather accept them as authoritative.

Communication Skills (unmet)

Margaret – your paper is very disjointed. Although some of the points you raise are important you do not discuss or analyse these with any depth or clarity. Your referencing is inaccurate throughout, and you have made many spelling and grammatical errors. Do come and talk with me about some strategies for improving your written communication.

Contribution to Group Learning (unmet)

You have not discussed this. Is that because there was no co-operation or collaboration?

Figure 8.3:   Examples of student feedback

In Figure 8.3 we offer examples of feedback at the three levels: 'well developed', 'developing' and 'unmet' for the assessment item discussed in Figure 8.3.

Students obviously find these comments helpful as the following student statements illustrate:

> *It is good to get feedback on your positive aspects and negative feedback helps you to acknowledge a problem and work towards improving it*

> *The only way you can learn how you are gaining in your learning, writing skills, group work*

> *Encouraged reflection and evaluation of self, group members' contributions, group dynamics, specific concepts.*

The examples above show responses to an individual assessment item, but even here students are encouraged to share their knowledge and to work collaboratively. Because nurses work closely with others it is important that the development of collaborative learning skills be encouraged throughout the course; assessment underlines the fact that such skills are seen as essential.

Group assessment

If students are to learn to work with each other then some assessment items need to be planned so that students produce work as a result of negotiation and co-operative learning. In such assignments the group as a whole will receive 'well developed', 'developing' or 'unmet' feedback. Such assessment items mean that students must plan how they will work together, and how they will deal with members who do not attend or contribute. They are continually encouraged to assess not only their own performance, but that of their peers. While this is very difficult for them initially, many groups become highly proficient at peer evaluation. Such proficiency is encouraged by facilitators paying frequent attention to how the group is working. Although group functioning is most commonly addressed informally it is included in formal assessment as explained above. Figure 8.4 shows an assessment sheet which assists the group to reflect informally on its own functioning.

Throughout the course a mix of individual and group assessment items is used, and students demonstrate great creativity in their group assessments. Such creativity is fostered by the opportunity for students to submit their assessment responses in various media. Sometimes they are asked to produce posters or models; at other times they are given the choice of the mode of presentation. An

Criteria for self/peer assessment	Well developed	Developing	Needs discussion
communicates openly;			
listens actively;			
respects the contributions of others;			
respects individual rights;			
assists in keeping the group on task;			
contributes to conflict resolution;			
supports group activities;			
contributes;			
information relevant to group learning goals;			
organises information for group use;			
seeks clarification of issues;			
participates in group feedback;			
reflects on own progress;			
evaluates self and peers' progress.			
Group assessment			
encourages shared responsibility;			
creates a supportive environment;			
respects individual's rights;			
recognises situations in need of improvement;			
gathers information effectively;			
identifies and works towards group learning goals;			
communicates ideas clearly;			
uses resources effectively;			
involves all group members.			

Figure 8.4:   Criteria for self, peer and group assessment

assessment item in Year 3 asked students, in groups, to present a situation where they had been required to be a client advocate. One group play-acted this situation with an angel and a devil representing aspects of the nurse's thinking, another group mimed the situation, another audio-taped an interview with an experienced nurse and yet others represented the situation with a series of video images.

In the first year, as part of a group assessment, students were asked to design a ward for family nursing. Some groups produced floor plans, others made flow charts and others produced models complete with curtains, floor coverings and paintings for the walls. We are often amazed by the ingenuity students demonstrate in their responses to group assignments; and students themselves tell us that they are a powerful and satisfying stimulus to learning.

When groups are planning their learning it is initially useful for them to identify who will do what. Figure 8.5 shows an example of a format designed to help students plan co-operative learning.

Such planning constitutes a learning contract which group members make with each other. Having ground rules, which the students develop for themselves, can be useful at the beginning of the course. For example, because some school leavers feel rather overawed by mature-aged students, and are rather reluctant to challenge

---

Group learning goals

Please list and provide a brief description of the learning goals identified by the group. Number each learning goal clearly.

1.
2.
3.
4.
5.
6.
7.
8.

Learning goal allocation

Please indicate which learning goal you have accepted. (More than one student may choose any given learning goal, but the learning goals should cover the important areas.)

Student name: . . . .   Learning Goal No: . . . .   Signature: . . . .
Student name: . . . .   Learning Goal No: . . . .   Signature: . . . .
Student name: . . . .   Learning Goal No: . . . .   Signature: . . . .
Student name: . . . .   Learning Goal No: . . . .   Signature: . . . .
Student name: . . . .   Learning Goal No: . . . .   Signature: . . . .
Student name: . . . .   Learning Goal No: . . . .   Signature: . . . .
Student name: . . . .   Learning Goal No: . . . .   Signature: . . . .
Student name: . . . .   Learning Goal No: . . . .   Signature: . . . .
Student name: . . . .   Learning Goal No: . . . .   Signature: . . . .
Student name: . . . .   Learning Goal No: . . . .   Signature: . . . .

Figure 8.5:   Group learning goals

or question, the group may need to establish some ways in which dialogue can be fostered. The group learning contract sets out each member's responsibilities to the group, and initially the facilitator may need to help the students in this process. Eventually, however, they tend to need neither the contracts nor the help of the facilitator in working out their group process.

Individual learning contracts

Individual learning contracts are the vehicle *par excellence* for enabling students to take control of, and assess, their own learning. The contract, which is a formal agreement between the student and the facilitator, will typically identify students' own learning goals, strategies to meet these, the criteria by which the achievement of learning goals will be measured and who will assess them. Often a registered nurse with whom the student will work is the nominated assessor, sometimes a peer, sometimes the university teacher, and sometimes the student will assess herself. Most commonly it is a mix of all of these. There is much satisfaction for students in being able to have control of their learning and to have this control taken seriously by teachers and clinical nurses. Such contracts can be used for either on- or off-campus learning. Figure 8.6 shows a student's learning goals for a three-week placement in a medical/surgical hospital ward.

---

1. To prioritise nursing care effectively throughout the shift.
2. To document effectively care given throughout the shift.
3. To give an informative and effective handover at the end of each shift.
4. To integrate relevant science concepts to nursing practice/skills.
5. To be competent in all areas of medication administration.
6. To enhance interpersonal communication skills, to facilitate effective assessments, implementation and evaluation of care plans and client education.
7. To develop and gain confidence in my clinical skills.
8. To identify all aspects of care involved in pre- and post-surgical clients.

Figure 8.6:   A Year 3 student's learning goals

The learning goals in Figure 8.6 were assessed, as the student had requested, by himself, his clinical preceptor and his university teacher. He developed criteria for each of his learning goals and gave them to the facilitator and the clinical preceptor before beginning his off-campus clinical experience. He indicated that he wished to be assessed as he would be on-campus, at a 'well developed', 'developing' or 'unmet' level.

Clinical assessment

Off-campus clinical assessment mirrors on-campus assessment. The use of some sort of learning contract always characterises assessment in the clinical area. Students are required to develop learning goals for each clinical placement, and to share these with the clinical teacher or preceptor. Clinical activities devised by the teaching team supplement the learning goals, and these activities are always related to the module which the students are currently working through. Three examples of clinical activities are given in Figure 8.7.

- This clinical activity requires you to give an oral presentation to your clinical group on a client you are caring for on this placement. You may wish to utilise the categories outlined below (Narrative Description, Significant Factors/Features, Situations in Need of Improvement, Hypothesis Testing, Clinical Judgement, Action Plan, Evaluation, Reflection) as a guide. Give your presentation to your clinical group in one of the afternoon debriefs. If you are in a community setting, organise to give your presentation to the facilitator and/or facility staff. In consultation with your facilitator, select a client whose situation reflects some of the modular concepts. (These are outlined at the end of the activity.) * Please note: this activity can be done in conjunction with your clinical aims, i.e. the same client can be used.

- Undertake a group process analysis of the team in the ward/area you have been allocated to. Utilise the group process assessment criteria used to evaluate group process at the university (see Figure 8.4). Share your intentions with staff in the area and also organise a time for staff to receive feedback.

- Medication Administration Activity – (This activity will not be possible in all settings. Negotiate with your facilitator to modify the activity if necessary). It is suggested that you undertake this activity in the first week of clinical to allow sufficient time for follow up.

  (i)   Develop criteria for self and facilitator evaluation of your oral medication administration skills.
  (ii) Negotiate with ward staff to administer oral medication to clients allocated to you. With your facilitator nominate times you wish to be evaluated (you may wish to include facility nursing staff in your evaluation). Write down times below.
  (iii) Self and facilitator and/or facility nursing staff evaluation.
  (iv) In the space below, reflect upon the activity and identify further learning needs and strategies for meeting these needs. Identify a time with your facilitator to review your progress.

Figure 8.7:   Clinical activities

On-campus clinical assessment takes place in the nursing laboratory. These experiences are discussed in earlier chapters but it may be useful to give some flavour of the major on-campus clinical assessment, the Global Nursing Practice Assessment (GNPA), here.

In the GNPA, one of which is incorporated in each year, students are given information about a range of clients with situations in need of improvement which they are likely to encounter in the assessment, covering learning issues and concepts which they will already have met in learning packages or in off-campus experiences. For one of these clients they will be expected to provide nursing care. Such care will always involve appropriate communication, and may range from the carrying out of a health assessment in Year 1, to the management of a person with multi-systems failure in Year 3. It may involve healthy clients who need education, or it may involve those with a psychiatric or physical illness, or both.

Assessment of their own performance is an integral part of the GNPA, and students are asked to bring a video-tape to record their interactions with the client. Subsequently they are asked to assess themselves and identify their strengths and weaknesses in the interaction.

A GNPA requires a large investment of teachers' time and resources, and usually takes place over one week, though the planning takes much longer. The teaching team decides upon the range of situations in need of improvement to be presented to students, and paid volunteers are trained to simulate this range of situations.

A typical GNPA might involve a number of discrete activities related to the client's situation. These could include the assessment of the client and the provision of some aspect of care; the documentation of that interaction; the presentation of a handover; some discussion of biological aspects of the person's situation such as the interpretation of pathology results or the pharmacodynamics of the client's medication regime; and finally an assessment of the interaction with the client as it is recorded on video-tape.

As with other assessments, the criteria for success in the GNPA are published in advance, and students are given detailed feedback both during and following the assessment.

Non-graded pass/fail

The decision about whether to grade students against each other or against specific criteria is not a difficult decision in problem-based learning. If we want co-operation and collaborative learning, then the way assessments are graded has strong influence on our ability to achieve. Some types of assessment are incompatible with, and counterproductive to, a problem-based approach to learning. In problem-based learning students are encouraged to be free to contribute to the whole process of learning. The students' developing abilities to do this are relatively fragile. We must therefore avoid everything which might discourage them from contributing to and valuing this contribution to their learning.

An assessment system where the mark becomes the reward, rather than the reward being the understanding of what students have learned and self-recognition of their learning skills, does not encourage learning for understanding; it promotes rote learning. A system which promotes competition, or is perceived to promote competition, will not foster co-operative learning, and will be perceived by both students and teachers to change the nature of the course. Non-graded pass/fail allows students to work together to produce individual work, or group work, knowing that it will be valued; it concentrates their attention on the comments explaining the 'well developed', 'developing' and 'unmet' under each criterion as the indication of their progress and achievements. A mix of individual and group assessment items helps to reinforce this, and Figure 8.8 shows a mix of assessment items in Year 1 and Year 3 of the course.

Many students come from an educational system which rewards individual competition and achievement, and some of them initially had difficulty with a system which valued co-operation and had a non-graded pass/fail system.

Year I Module I – Health, Culture and Care

1. *Presentation on nursing roles and functions*

   – after reading, viewing videos and interviewing nurses in various roles in the community and in hospital, students will present their findings to facilitators and the group.

2. *A group presentation of a poster* of any aspect of adolescent sexuality for use by a school health nurse as a teaching strategy within high schools. Poster to include any key set of core concepts (physical, social, environmental, psychological)
   – after reading, talking with adolescents and school health nurses, students, as a group, will prepare a poster for presentation to the total group.

3. *Publishing findings of a health assessment in the student newspaper*

   – as a group, students will carry out health assessment of the university community and, using a comparative external sample, will publish their results in the student newspaper.

4. *A study of a migrant family*

   – students will be required to select a migrant family and make an assessment of it in terms of: – family roles, socio-economic status, health beliefs, health behaviours, child-rearing practices and activities of living.

Year 3 Module I – Complex Health Breakdown I

1. *Group presentation and group written presentation of the concept of crisis in relation to nursing practice*

   – students will choose a client situation in which a crisis occurred for the client or family and consider the nurse's role and mode of intervention. In groups of 4 present the situation (role-play, audio-visual, story-telling, audio-tape, written) to the rest of your university group. This will incorporate discussion of your group process. Analyse the factors which have an impact on the nurse/client situation and present this in a written form. You need to consider the concept of crisis in relation to nursing practice and may need to examine such issues as the nature of the situation, personal and professional values and beliefs, etc., along with responsibilities involved and their relevance for intervention on strategies.

2. *Individual clinical assessment*

   – during your clinical placement select an acutely ill client with whom you are actively involved in assessing, planning, implementing and evaluating holistic care. Negotiate with your clinical facilitator/preceptor to present a situation improvement summary for this client for assessment/feedback. Also negotiate with your clinical facilitator/preceptor opportunities for her/him to observe your nursing practice of this client for an extended period to allow for the provision of evaluative feedback.

3. *Individual assessment: addressing a client's community*

   – choose one of the clients you actively cared for during your clinical placement with the aim of making an analysis of this person's community. Make a thorough analysis of this person's community (family, significant others, social services, community supports, welfare agencies, etc.) and the impact which this has on his/her health status. The assessment will include discussions with the client, family and various caregivers and community services. How effective is the person's community in supporting the person after discharge and preventing re-admission? What elements impinge upon the effectiveness of the community (eg. policy issues at local, state and commonwealth government level; the person's knowledge of available services; education in the use of services; access and availability of services, etc.)?

Figure 8.8:   Mixture of group/individual items, Years I & 3

I found it difficult the first year coming from school and everything there was competitive, especially in year 12. You have to get that TE [Tertiary Entrance] score, you have to be better than the next person. Coming into an environment where you work as a group and you just throw everything on the table, I found that for a while I wouldn't speak a lot in the group and I wouldn't give much to it because I thought I was disadvantaging myself – and then I started looking at it, and I realised it was more of an advantage because you work as a group and you do group assignments, but it was difficult. From listening to other people's courses they say 'How come you just hand over the information like that – that's good stuff, you could have used that for your assignment?' Well, we all do it, everyone. If you've got something that's going to help understand that particular thing better then you just scoot it over and say 'Here you go, try it that way.'

Kimberly, Year 3 student

It has been our experience that students are not inhibited by a pass/fail system from doing their best work. On the contrary, students take immense pride in the fact that they have been able to have responsibility for their own learning.

I think if everyone was graded it would change the whole atmosphere of the place.

Carmela, Year 3 student

It [grading] would change the whole idea of problem-based learning.

Orlando, Year 3 student

Exit profiles

If a non-graded pass/fail assessment system is used, then the individual academic transcript gives little information about the student other than that they have achieved a non-graded pass or a fail. The transcript can be amplified by a student exit profile which mirrors the assessment feedback sheets, and gives valuable information to potential employers, or to institutions where students might wish to undertake further study. It provides information related to the four assessment categories used in the course. An example of such a document is shown in Figure 8.9.

Student exit profile

Student Name: Ursula Fowler

This exit profile reflects the extent to which the above student has met the course aims (see below). Evaluation and assessment of student ability by faculty, peers and self is integral to the course.

Course Aims:

The course will prepare graduates who practise facilitative care which:
* *promotes client self-care
* *enables and empowers clients to resolve problems of health care
* *synthesises experience – practice – theory
* *incorporates a critical approach to all professional behaviour
* *is enhanced by self reflection in that practice
* *contributes to the knowledge, attitudes, values and skill base of the profession

The course aims are matched with the Australasian Nurses Registering Authorities' Competencies, so that students who satisfy the course requirements have automatically met those competency standards.

Assessment throughout the course is on the basis of the criteria categories used below to outline this student's achievements.

Assessment Categories

1. *Concepts and theories*

This category covers the extent to which this student has demonstrated the ability to identify and apply an appropriate range of concepts and theories across a variety of situations.

> Ursula consistently demonstrated highly developed analytical skills, synthesising and applying an appropriate range of concepts/theories across a variety of situations. Her work is thorough and thoughtful. Analyses of clinical situations have been client-centred and have reflected a comprehensive and holistic approach to care. Clinical feedback indicated that Ursula's application of nursing skills was of a high quality.

2. *Utilisation of resources*

This category covers the extent to which this student has demonstrated the ability to find and use relevant information and ideas from formal sources (eg. books) and informal sources (eg. knowledgeable people).

> Ursula is interested in understanding as many facets of a situation as possible. Thus, she has effectively accessed, integrated and used a wide range of information from a variety of sources both on-campus and during clinical experiences.

3. *Communication skills*

This category covers this student's written communication as it relates to appropriate academic writing standards and interpersonal communication skills as they relate to off-campus client care and on-campus tutorials.

> Ursula's written skills are effective. Work is clearly expressed and well-structured demonstrating an appropriate academic standard. Interpersonal skills with clients and colleagues are effective. Ursula articulates her ideas in a clear and cogent manner, she is an interested listener and engages easily in discussion.

4. *Contribution to group enquiry process*

Students learn co-operatively in small group processes throughout the course. This category covers this student's ability to contribute and work collaboratively in a group setting.

> Ursula made a substantial contribution to group learning activities. She is a highly motivated and self-directed person and demonstrates effective group skills.

Figure 8.9:   Example of an exit profile

Conclusion

In examining the role assessment plays within a problem-based learning course, this chapter has outlined the ways in which we have used assessment to help students to learn and the ways in which individual and group assessments both on- and off-campus have been structured to encourage and promote creative and integrated learning. The system of criterion-referenced assessment describes how this is used to evaluate and respond to students' work. In using a non-graded pass/fail assessment system the importance of facilitator, peer and self-assessment is discussed with examples used to illustrate how the issues are addressed. Twenty-five years ago it was common to find statements that assessment had the dual purpose of accreditation (rewarding assessment) and encouraging learning. The obvious failure of assessment systems to achieve the latter resulted in this idea falling from the agenda; we have shown how, in a problem-based course, it is achieved.

Chapter 9
The role of evaluation

Don Margetson

Excellent chance to comment and therefore play a part in making future changes for future students.

Yvonne, student

Evaluation is often thought of quite separately from the design and implementation of a course of study; on this view, it is the third element which may or may not be added after design and implementation have been completed. In contrast, we take an integrated view consistent with the nature of problem-based learning. In this chapter we discuss the importance of evaluation in facing up to assumptions, knowledge and value explicitly throughout the design and implementation of a course, as well as in the more familiar sense concerned with outcomes of a course at particular times.

The integrated view of evaluation taken in a problem-based course acknowledges the pervasive presence of evaluation in human action and understanding. In earlier chapters we have seen how this is reflected in problem-based learning itself – for example, in student evaluations of hypotheses about a case they are studying, of the quality of information used in reaching tentative decisions, of the plan of action they develop for the purpose of improving the situation under consideration and of how well a plan of action might work in practice. While these examples are taken from nursing, similar activities would be found in any problem-based learning course. Their significance is easily underestimated.

Far from being merely incidental details of problem-based student learning, the integration of evaluation into learning counters the larger issue of the fragmentation of knowledge into isolated specialisms which pervades virtually all aspects of life. A serious consequence for education has been the tendency to restrict evaluation to a narrow specialised role quite separate from the design and implementation of a course of study.

Midgley (1991) points to the deep need for education to take stock of where it stands currently and where it is going. Problem-based learning is well positioned on this question. It has already, in systematic educational practice, begun to overcome the debilitating belief in an absolute gap between fact and value. Year 3 students were well aware of the nature of evaluation as integral in human activity and of the necessity for specific evaluation activities:

> *I ... realise they are necessary to make improvements. Evaluation is needed everywhere, even in personal life.*
>
> Amy, Year 3 student

The following example illustrates Amy's point. Suppose students were studying the level of health in a community, and that hypothesis A – concerned with hygienic water supply, social support structures and the like – explained the level of health better than did hypothesis B which was concerned with patterns of visits to health practitioners. In terms of the belief in an absolute fact/value split, this situation would seem to have to do with facts and not values. In one way of course it does: if certain organisms are present in the water supply people will die from drinking the water, and that is appropriately described as a fact rather than a value. But it is not simply a question of either fact or value.

For it is also a fact that we do not take all facts to be equally valuable, and we tend to act accordingly. Some facts are typically regarded as more important than others, and this is itself an expression of value that we take seriously and act upon. That a hygienic community water supply, for example, is more important than reducing the price of cinema tickets expresses the value that it is generally good for persons to be biologically healthy and that, whatever other physical, mental, emotional or spiritual goods and benefits we may seek, a hygienic water supply normally has a crucial place in supporting the health of persons. Consequently, communities which understand and are in a position to do something about hygienic water supply take extensive action to ensure its provision. The central place of value in human action and understanding illustrated by this example has two specific implications for problem-based learning.

The first is that the place of evaluation as an integral part of student learning is made quite explicit in problem-based learning. Evaluating situations – whether theoretical or practical, professional or academic – is an important part of any learning. Without evaluation, particularly in the form of reflective evaluation on what is to be or, later, has been learned, how it has been learned and for what purpose, learners can easily lose their way in a mass of seemingly unrelated information.

The second is that in principle the same kinds of questions apply just as much to the design and implementation of any course of study, although there will be specific aspects distinctive of different areas of study. Overall evaluative questions in the case of nursing, for example, include: is such and such a way of preparing nurses at the undergraduate level likely to be as effective as alternative ways, by what standards are judgements made, who is affected by decisions made, what are the implications of these decisions for communities affected by the decisions, and so on? Questions such as these are not always easy to get to grips with and to resolve.

In a word, they can be problematic. This implies that the design of a course of study, just like the learning which students undertake in a problem-based course, is itself a problem-based activity in which evaluation is an integral, constitutive part. Although there is an important role for discrete, if rare, external evaluations of a course, in general evaluation is not merely a disconnected activity which can, optionally, be adopted at occasional intervals.

For any group establishing a problem-based course, whether this be from scratch or transforming a more traditional course, it is therefore important to consider the place of evaluation from the very beginning. The problem-based nursing course at Griffith University provides an example of this in practice.

Evaluation in the design of the course

The crucial importance of evaluation emerged early in the design of the course. Following Griffith University's decision in principle to introduce a course in nursing, the Vice-Chancellor established a Nursing Studies Planning Group to carry forward the planning for such a course. The Planning Group met for the first time in October 1988, and invited nursing consultants from two other higher education institutions, a representative of nursing from the Queensland Health Department and a representative of the university's higher education centre (the present author) to join it at its second meeting in November 1988.

Up until the second meeting of the group, a nursing course had been thought of mainly as an extension to the activities of the Faculty of Science and Technology. The faculty had proposed an essentially applied physical and biological sciences model of nursing, although some time later alternative ideas for a new faculty to include nursing, chiropractic and applied behavioural sciences had been floated elsewhere in the university. The applied sciences model of nursing was reflected in a submission by the Faculty of Science and Technology to the Queensland Minister for Health which acknowledged the relevance of such studies as 'sociology and health care' to nursing but emphasised the faculty's 'well recognised role in medical research'. The submission conceived of nursing in entirely hospital-based terms in that a central aim of the intended course was to produce 'highly trained and educated professional nursing staff to meet the demand for such staff in hospitals located in the southern Brisbane-Gold Coast region' (Griffith University 1988a). Widening the membership of the Group to include relevant expertise brought different views to bear.

Bringing evaluation into planning

The evaluation of current and projected needs of nursing education provided by the consultants at the second meeting of the planning group was very different from the applied physical and biological sciences model of nursing. The consultants indicated that, while there would always be a place for 'high-tech' nursing in special hospital settings to which a science faculty's medical research interests would be relevant, nursing could not sensibly be restricted to such a narrow role. As the meeting agreed, 'nursing sciences includ[ed] relevant aspects of the behavioural, social, biological and physical sciences' but also encompassed, for example, 'the promotion of health, prevention of illness, health teaching and care of physically and mentally ill and disabled people, of all ages and in all health care and community settings' (Griffith University 1988b).

Starting from this position, the planning group developed its conception of an appropriate course over a number of meetings between November 1988 and June 1989. This phase of planning culminated in a document entitled 'Nursing Studies: Development of Planning' (Margetson 1989b), and illustrates the central importance of evaluation in planning. The initial version of the document was organised under four main headings: Conception; Design Requirements; Indication of Curriculum Forms; and Timetable for Planning. Questions were asked, under Design Requirements in particular, about the purpose of nursing and how it functions. This helped avoid the assumption that ready-made answers from existing practices in other areas of study were necessarily the best available for nursing. The questions kept open, quite explicitly, the possibility of making use of the best features of existing knowledge, understanding and practice, but understood and structured in relation to the purposes of a degree course in nursing. From answers to these questions, the document drew conclusions about requirements for learning, teaching and the curriculum. At each meeting of the planning group during this phase the content of the document was evaluated and developed with the result that it evolved through several cycles to reach its final articulation in the fourth version of the document.

Evaluation is a necessary part of articulating a conception of a course of study so that more detailed planning can follow coherently. Without a conception articulated in some detail a planning group will be proceeding somewhat in the dark, confusion and misunderstandings are more probable within the group and for those joining the course later, and without systematic evaluation both flaws and creative design opportunities in a conception are likely to be missed.

Evaluating curriculum implications

In regard to the curriculum, this meant that an evaluative question concerning design was confronted explicitly: were some forms of curriculum likely to be better than others in achieving the course aim – that is, high-quality professional nurses who would be able to practise effectively in the context identified under Design Requirements? But this raises a general difficulty of evaluation in the design of any new curriculum and of any curriculum change – and equally for any decision *not* to change. That is, while it is desirable to base curriculum decisions on comprehensive evaluation of curricula in comparable situations, such evaluations are not always available. In the case of the proposed nursing activity, no comprehensive evaluations of problem-based nursing courses were available since no such courses were known. How, then, could sound decisions be reached; if complete, formal, systematic evaluation results are not available, does this mean that decisions must be merely subjective?

Not at all, for at least two reasons. First, informed critical judgement needs to be brought to bear in evaluating an innovative proposal in this as in any area. Second, a growing literature exists particularly in a health-related field, namely medicine, where evaluative information is available from fully problem-based medical courses such as those at McMaster University in Canada, Newcastle University in Australia and the Rijksuniversiteit Limburg, in Maastricht, the Netherlands, as well as in higher education more generally (see the bibliography at the end of the book for some references). Since better and worse evaluative judgements can be made depending on the quality of evidence and thought which goes into reaching a judgement, the planning group worked systematically towards identifying which form of curriculum would be most likely to lead to the desired outcome.

Dealing with controversy in evaluation at the design stage

The absence of directly comparable evaluative information from other courses in this case also illustrates how large evaluation questions are seldom amenable to simple yes/no, good/bad, answers, and that evaluation is typically a complex matter. Consequently, the design of any new course of study can be expected to involve controversy. In the planning of the nursing course, dispute focused on the main alternatives under consideration – effectively, the applied science model on the one hand and the independent nursing-focused model on the other. Apart from the usual political aspects such as faculties seeking to extend their influence, more fundamental questions of understanding arise. A sociologist, say, will have come to value the knowledge provided by sociology, just as a physicist will have come to value the knowledge provided by physics, and both are, in good faith, likely to read their values into situations they know little about. Thus the physicist may take it as 'natural' that a nursing course could be valuable only if it adhered to an applied science model, while the sociologist might be equally convinced that the course would be valuable only if students in it constructed their own realities. These evaluations are central to the views taken by the respective individuals, but in many conventional planning situations they remain tacit and unexamined.

In contrast to this, the design process followed in the Griffith case centred on an explicitly articulated conception of the activity which brought values out, went to some lengths to resolve differences between them constructively and made clear the implications of the conception and its justification for the design of the activity. This has implications for the amount of time to be devoted to design activity and the evaluation of design proposals (Boud and Feletti 1991:56), as well as for institutional commitment (Little and Sauer 1991). It also has implications for the staff development activity we have discussed in Chapter 7, particularly in relation to providing a clear articulation of the activity for staff subsequently joining the course.

The result of such a process in the case of the Griffith nursing course was that the planning group reached the view that nursing is related to a number of disciplines, not only to biological sciences, and that 'nursing as an autonomous profession benefited from links with a range of academic activities' (Griffith University 1989).

In summary, then, what can we say about the importance of evaluation at the design stage for the planning of any problem-based course? The central lesson illustrated by this case is that without systematic evaluation of a coherently evolving conception, effective design of a proposed course of study is in real danger of being short-circuited. Specific dangers to adequate planning and design include unevaluated assumptions that:

- knowledge must be fragmented, and that fragments must necessarily coincide with existing divisions;
- existing curriculum arrangements in an institution will be suitable for a new academic activity;
- narrow views from existing academic activities in an institution need not be evaluated but can simply be acted upon;
- existing power-groupings pursuing their own legitimate self-interests will in all respects take decisions which are in the best interests of the new activity.

Conversely, the case illustrates the importance of planning and design structures and processes which incorporate evaluation as a vital and integral activity; these include:

- a clearly identified planning group with a specific brief to evaluate the variety of course-design options available;
- inclusion of relevant expertise in the planning group, including expertise from outside the institution where necessary;
- articulation, in some depth, of a coherent overall conception of the proposed activity and its requirements in regard to teaching and learning (from undergraduate level through to postgraduate research), curriculum, location in the institutional structure, relations to related activities both inside and outside the institution, and administration;
- appointment to the proposed activity, at the earliest stage possible, of academic staff – including the person who is to head the activity – clearly in sympathy with the conception of the proposed activity and committed to its evolving implementation in practice;
- adequate time and support for thorough planning.

Evaluation of the course in operation

Consistent with the principle of including evaluation as an integral part of problem-based learning, the course has itself been systematically evaluated in operation, primarily for formative purposes. Evaluative information has been gathered in ways ranging from the comparatively formal (the first five items below) to the informal. These include:

- a survey of the class as a whole on their reaction to the course on two occasions during the first year the course was run (1991), and a similar survey of staff on the first occasion;
- surveys of each problem-based student group on its own response to a learning package;
- surveys of students during their clinical placements;
- interviews of third-year students nearing the end of their course (extracts from which have been given in this book), and parallel interviews of staff;
- two surveys of these third-year students, using, first, a questionnaire drawn up by members of the teaching team, and, second, a questionnaire used in national surveys;
- approximately monthly meetings of a staff co-ordinator and student representatives from each problem-based tutorial group;
- open forums from time to time (usually stemming from the meetings of co-ordinator and student representatives) when students felt there was a need to discuss issues more widely;
- a deliberate seeking out by staff of feedback from students, especially during third year, of views on the course.

The responsiveness of staff to students' evaluative views, gathered in the ways described above, played an important part in the success of the course. Although students occasionally found regular evaluation questionnaires on learning packages somewhat tedious, students generally appreciated the opportunity to give their views:

> *Glad we get them, so we can air our grievances.*
>
> *Tonya, Year 3 student*

Staff responsiveness was important individually, through informal staff and student groups, and through more formal processes, such as the reporting of survey results to an evaluation sub-committee of the committee responsible for running the course. Students often feel affirmed when their thoughts and opinions are taken seriously – particularly when changes to the course and practices within it take place as a result of careful consideration of their feedback – and this can have a very encouraging and positive effect on their studies.

Other evaluative information was of course available too. The normal assessment of written work by students, student performance in GNPAs and the experiences encountered by facilitators in their classes (problem-based tutorials, laboratories, etc.) provide a rich source of evaluative information for critical consideration.

Information from the overall surveys was distributed both to teaching teams and to students. The teaching teams used this information in regular meetings to consider whether any changes should be made to the course. In addition, individual members of a teaching team used the information in considering their own teaching activities in the course, largely as facilitators of problem-based student groups. Towards the end of the course, in the third year, students were surveyed for their views of the whole course as they had experienced it. Below, we will consider these matters in more detail, beginning with descriptions of the survey methods and main results. Then, in a section on 'Effect on the course' we will consider some examples of how evaluation has affected the course.

Survey methods: student responses to learning packages

At the end of each learning package each facilitator had the option of routinely distributing to her problem-based student group a standard questionnaire on one sheet of paper. The processes of collecting completed questionnaires, obtaining results and distributing results to those concerned is described in more detail in Appendix 8 together with an example of results and the covering note to the facilitator drawing attention to some important information about the results.

Responses to each learning package varied from group to group, as could be expected where styles of facilitation and group work varied considerably. Student responses often referred to quite detailed matters that could be reasonably interpreted only by the facilitator of the group, as the following example – a verbatim student response listed under 'Best features' – indicates: 'Urine testing – re: "Miracle of Life" video'. This kind of feedback was found by facilitators to be useful in their conduct of subsequent learning packages, and towards the end of semester when learning packages were reviewed systematically by the whole teaching team. Similar remarks apply to the clinical feedback. An example of how results of student evaluation affected the course is given later in the section entitled 'Effect on the course'.

Survey methods: student views of facilitation

Some evaluative information on their facilitation was gained by individual facilitators through the learning package evaluation questionnaires. However, such information was incidental to the main purpose, which was to gather information on student perceptions of the learning package. In order to gain more systematic information on their facilitation, some facilitators in fact used the learning package questionnaire and students were asked to comment on facilitation rather than on the package. The same processing arrangement as is described in Appendix 8 for the learning package evaluation was used.

A questionnaire specifically designed to gather information on facilitation was also developed, with results returned to the facilitator concerned. A copy of the questionnaire is given in Appendix 9.

Survey methods: the clinical experience

Students and facilitators (both university and clinical facilitators) responded to their experience of the clinical placement aspects of the course. Responses were obtained by questionnaire similar in form to that used for student responses to learning packages. Unlike the process for learning package responses (where completed student questionnaires were processed independently of the teaching team and the results, reported in a generalised form which did not reveal the identities of students, for each group forwarded to the member of the teaching team for her problem-based group), completed clinical questionnaires were returned by students directly to the clinical co-ordinator who circulated them to the external agencies concerned and to the facilitators. Evaluative information relating to clinical experience has been discussed in detail in Chapter 6.

Survey methods: Year 3 surveys

Towards the end of their course of studies, in the second semester of the third year, students were surveyed by two different questionnaires. One questionnaire was drawn up by members of the teaching team, the other, a Course Experience Questionnaire (Ramsden 1992), was a standard instrument that has been used in large-scale national surveys.

The questionnaires were thus complementary. The first provided information on particular aspects of the course on which the teaching team wanted feedback, the second provided a measure of comparability between student responses to this particular problem-based nursing course and a broad background of student responses to a wider variety of degree courses in different contexts. The value of such a broad comparison is that it gives some idea of whether a problem-based course is within the range of student responses to studies in general. Clearly, if the responses to a problem-based course were significantly worse than could be expected generally in courses of study, then there would be cause for serious concern; conversely, a significantly better response would be encouraging, although identifying factors making for either of these situations would require a great deal of further investigation.

In the event, the Year 3 survey results gave cause for considerable optimism about the Griffith course as it was experienced by the first cohort of students to complete the course. Main results of the Course Experience Questionnaire are given in Figure 9.1, together with comparable results from a national survey which was conducted during the time the nursing course was running.

Results of individual items in the Course Experience Questionnaire are not as reliable as the scales given in Figure 9.1 which combine a number of related items. However, very strong mean responses for an individual item may suggest something worth noting. Taking (arbitrarily) values of mean responses of about 50 or above and of about −50 or below as 'very strong', ten responses out of the forty-three items in the questionnaire stand out. These are listed in Figure 9.2. All may be interpreted as identifying favourable aspects of the course; no unfavourable aspects gained very strong responses as defined. Note that items attracting a *low* mean on the original score which indicated a *favourable* response (i.e., items 8, 26, 12, 25 in Figure 9.2) have here had their phrasing 'reversed' so as to preserve the intended meaning in the transform scoring system, i.e., the statement of the item has been preceded by the phrase 'It is false that'.

Survey methods: open forums

Occasionally, at the request of students, open forums of staff and students were held to discuss issues of concern to students. The forums were chaired by a member of staff, but often students nominated the member of staff to chair a forum. Forums focused on issues which the students particularly wanted to discuss.

	Griffith (Nathan)[1] course		National survey[2] nursing (initial)[3]		National survey all fields of study	
	Mean.	sd	Mean.	sd	Mean.	sd
Appropriate assessment	49[4]	37	32	39	37	43
Good teaching	34	36	4	37	6	40
Appropriate workload	27	42	−9	38	3	40
Emphasis on student independence	24	32	Not available			
Clear goals and standards	−4	43	2	39	14	40
The following is a single item, not a scale						
Overall satisfaction with the course	34	64	18	51	32	51

Figure 9.1:   Results of Course Experience Questionnaire, and some national comparisons

Notes

1. Griffith University has two schools, on different campuses, offering nursing. The course referred to here is only the initial Bachelor of Nursing course on the Nathan campus of Griffith University. The number of students responding to the Course Experience Questionnaire was forty-three (approximately a third of the final year group).

2. Long, Michael (1993) *Course Experience Questionnaire, 1992 Graduates*, Australian Council for Educational Research. Numbers of students responding: nursing (initial): just under 2700; all fields of study: around 52,500 (numbers responding to different items fluctuated slightly; e.g. the number of responses for all fields of study varied between 52,434 and 52,568).

3. In the national survey students were surveyed some months after completing their initial, i.e., pre-registration, courses of study. The Griffith students were surveyed late in their course, at the point when their studies were almost completed.

4. An explanation of the numerical values is as follows. Scoring on the Course Experience Questionnaire used the response scale 1 'strongly disagree' to 5 'strongly agree'. In the national survey, results were transformed into values ranging from −100 to +100 including 'reversing' values where appropriate (e.g., a questionnaire item 'Staff here show no real interest in what students have to say' attracting a mean response of 1.0 would be a very *favourable* response since it expresses strong disagreement with the item. Therefore in the transform this would be interpreted as 'staff here show a real interest in what students have to say' and would be represented as a value of 100, not −100). The correspondence is as follows:

$$1 = -100; 2 = -50; 3 = 0; 4 = 50; 5 = 100.$$

Questionnaire Item no.		Mean
Section 1: The course in general		
9	The course seems to encourage us to develop our own academic interests	50
15	The staff make a real effort to understand difficulties students may be having with their work	50
17	Teaching staff here normally give helpful feedback on how you are going	50
8	[It is false that] To do well on this course all you really need is a good memory	65
26	[It is false that] It would be possible to get through this course just by working hard around exam times	65
12	[It is false that] Staff here seem more interested in testing what we've memorised than what we've understood	60
25	[It is false that] Staff here show no real interest in what students have to say	50
Section 2: Studying the course material		
38	In trying to understand new ideas, I often try to relate them to real life situations to which they might apply	60
32	I try to relate ideas in this subject to those in others, wherever possible	55
33	I usually set out to understand thoroughly the meaning of what I am asked to read	50

Figure 9.2: Items attracting strong responses in the Course Experience Questionnaire, Year 3 students, Griffith University

For example, at a Year 2 Forum, in Semester 1, 1992, issues raised included clinical placements and facilitation; university facilitation; assessment; and learning packages. The forum followed a process of students in small groups identifying what they considered to be positive and negative about each of these issues, and what changes they thought would be desirable. Items from small groups were pooled for the whole group to see, and an indication taken from each group as to whether it thought the positives outweighed the negatives, or vice versa, or were evenly balanced. Feedback from these forums supports the view expressed in Chapter 7 that a crucially important element in the success of a problem-based course is adequate orientation for new staff integrated with an ongoing process of staff development. The 1992 Year 2 forum illustrates this. Some of the student concerns arose from perceptions of inadequate facilitation during that year (e.g., students commented that there was 'Too much guess work' in dealing with learning packages and that the packages 'reflect facilitators' personal interests') and with related matters reflecting an apparently poor understanding of the nature of the course by some staff (e.g., students commented that 'Facilitators need to be aware of philosophy of course', and that facilitation needed to be 'Less judgemental' and give 'more direction').

These perceptions contrast with student perceptions of the facilitation provided by those staff more experienced in problem-based teaching and in the nature of a problem-based course. The picture is complicated by factors which would not be specifically to do with problem-based learning (e.g., student comments included 'Hospital staff unaware of student activities', 'Labs need more direction', 'Anti-male feeling', 'Expectations [of different staff] inconsistent' and 'Lack of communication'). However, there is sufficient information specifically to do with problem-based learning, and enough of that information which draws attention to the need for staff development on facilitation and the nature of problem-based courses in particular, to make the student perceptions obtained in forums very useful. An example of the way in which feedback from an open forum affected subsequent running of the course is discussed later in the section entitled 'Effect on the course'.

Survey methods: Year 1 student views of the course as a whole

Twice during the first year in which the course was run (1991), a little after mid-semester, student and teaching team responses to the course as a whole were obtained by means of a form of nominal group technique. It will be useful to describe this process in order to illustrate in some detail how an evaluation process provided formative feedback to the teaching team in one semester so that appropriate improvements could be made in the following semester. Details are given in Appendix 9; here we will summarise the main results.

The number of Year 1 students responding to the first of the surveys of the course as a whole (conducted on 7 May 1991, during the tenth week of teaching) was 145, which represented 78 per cent of the students enrolled in the course. The number of staff (i.e., the teaching team) responding was ten. The main results (top five items) are summarised in Figure 9.3.

Perhaps the most striking (though not surprising) result was that, independently, both staff and students ranked 'Large group numbers' as the worst feature of the course, and both gave 'Smaller groups' as the most desirable change. (Each problem-based student group comprises around eighteen to twenty students. This may be compared with typical problem-based medical courses, where the equivalent groups comprise around seven to eight students (Engel 1991). The large group size in nursing is largely a result of current financial stringency affecting universities.)

It is important to note that the statements resulting from the surveys were not necessarily taken as conclusive by themselves, and that this principle applied

	1st priority	2nd priority	3rd priority	4th priority	5th priority
Students *Best features*	Problems in problem-based learning.	The clinical week.	No exams (and, equally ranked) Having a facilitator to ourselves.	Given the two repetitions of exams, it may be useful to note the two statements next highest in rank i.e. Being in small groups promotes more interactions between group members; and you learn more because you research it yourself and therefore you retain more information (and, equally ranked) Group interaction.	No exams.
Staff *Best features*	The student is at the centre of the learning process.	Learning is structured in a relevant context.	Communication and group building are integral components of the learning experience.	Nursing is a central theme in the course.	Nursing is a central theme in the course.
Students *Worst features*	Large group numbers.	Lack of facilitator guidance.	Lectures should be more structured; direct information should be given out and lecture notes should be printed and not in running writing (and, equally ranked) X's lectures (personal names mentioned by students were replaced by 'X', and the student comment forwarded in confidence only to the person named).	The availability, accessibility and amount of resources are limited.	Lack of information in regard to, for example, the library.

	1st priority	2nd priority	3rd priority	4th priority	5th priority
Staff *Worst features*	Large group numbers.	Facilitation is exhausting.	Emotional strain when the group process breaks down.	Student groups are isolated from each other and from other facilitators.	There are so many areas that need definition or re-addressing and there is so little time and energy to do (and, equally ranked) The amount of planning/ preparation of second semester while teaching in first semester.
Students *Changes*	Smaller groups.	More direct links with hospitals.	More structure for first year or even part of it.	More practical skills.	Give students a better idea about what they have to learn.
Staff *Changes*	Smaller groups.	Follow through on team-building to allow constructive criticism as well as positive comments.	Revise pacing.	More time (and equally ranked) Opportunity for facilitators to learn from each other.	Some weeks without learning packages trying other self-directed methods.

Figure 9.3: Main results of first survey: top five items produced by students and staff, in descending order of priority

to all evaluative information. For example, as noted above in the student view, the second worst feature of the course was 'Lack of facilitator guidance'. This perception needs careful consideration. Does it mean (a) that facilitators were giving too little guidance – inadequate facilitation, in effect? If so, then it would seem that the facilitators concerned would need to consider ways of facilitating more effectively. But it might not mean this; it might mean (b) that students who were, at high school perhaps, used to being talked at in a more didactic mode were seeking a return to what they were used to. Were they, in effect, expressing dislike of a learning process that required them to be much more active and to think for themselves? If this is what is meant by their statement that there was a 'Lack of facilitator guidance', then it is not at all clear that the *appropriate* response by facilitators would be simply to provide more 'instruction'.

Let us now consider some examples of how results from this and other surveys of student and staff perceptions of the course as a whole affected subsequent activity in the course.

Effect on the course

Action in the light of evaluation: the processing framework

A clear example of action taken in the light of the evaluative information gathered in the survey of Year 1 student views of the course as whole is the following. Some students had commented that a worst feature of the course was 'Gaps between lectures' (referring to the fact that there was no formal tutorial class contact from late Monday afternoon to Wednesday morning in a typical week).

If students perceived a 'gap' between classes as a waste of time, and perceived problem-based tutorials as 'lectures', then what conception of the course did students have? In fact this perceived 'gap' was designed into the course as an integral part of the learning process. This time was set aside for students to seek out and learn the material they needed to know in order to deal with the problems they had identified in their analysis of situations in need of improvement. That analysis was carried out during problem-based tutorials on a Monday. In the light of what they had learned before the problem-based tutorial on the Wednesday, students would, in the Wednesday class, pool, discuss and evaluate what they had learned in order to further their understanding of the matter being studied (see page 14 for an outline of the timetable). Some students seemed not to have grasped points such as these about the learning process central to problem-based learning.

In response to this, the teaching team developed a processing framework for use by facilitators and students. The development of the processing framework is itself an example of problem-based learning in action, in this case on the part of staff. In the terms used in the course, evaluation of activity revealed a situation in need of improvement, the situation was analysed and appropriate action taken in the light of it. The processing framework itself, just over two pages in length, comprised 'some crucial questions' together with 'some useful prompts' – e.g., 'Is there a situation in need of improvement? – analyse the data; identify cues'; if there is a situation in need of improvement, or more than one, 'What are your possible explanations for these situations? – list tentative hypotheses; which are the most likely hypotheses'; and 'What do you need to know in order to confirm or reject these explanations? – list learning needs' (the processing framework is given in full in Appendix 1).

As far as students were concerned, some encouraging responses in Semester 2 were received in regard to the use of this framework. This type of response was reiterated by Year 3 students (see, for example, Appendix 10 which includes the item: 'Being able to apply the clinical reasoning skills used in processing learning packages.' This item received the high mean score of student responses of 4.1 on a scale of 0–5, with 5 representing 'Very useful'). Other evaluative feedback has revealed the difficulty that some students (and even some facilitators) see the processing framework as too mechanistic and restrictive – a risk clearly foreseen by the group who developed the framework. In fact, because of the risk, considerable discussion had taken place as to whether the processing framework should be developed at all. On balance, the view was taken that it would be helpful since students and staff in the course were clearly in need of some support in this direction. It was emphasised to all staff that the processing framework was not to be seen as a rigid mechanism to be followed blindly; indeed, it was suggested that it be regarded more as a kind of temporary crutch to be thrown away as soon as it was no longer needed. None the less, in some cases the processing framework has been regarded and used in a way quite the opposite of that intended.

This reinforces the point, already mentioned, of the importance in early design work of producing a clearly articulated conception of the proposed course. This alone, however, is not enough. A thoroughly articulated conception of an academic activity clearly set out in a document also needs to be used. Such a document has to be incorporated in a staff development process involving ongoing discussion and active participation by staff, as discussed in Chapter 7. This process, as an integral part of the development of a course in the light of systematic evaluation, cannot be adequately characterised as 'training'. It goes well beyond mere training in that it necessarily involves reflection on practice, openness to an enriched understanding of the course under consideration and critical evaluation of the course in operation as well as the original conception.

The last point – evaluation of the conception in comparison with the experience of a course in operation – is vital. The relation is not one-way. That is, this evaluation cannot be interpreted satisfactorily as starting with an unchangeably fixed conception to which experience has to conform – equally, it is not a case simply of fixed experience totally determining changes to the conception. The relation is deeper, more complex and subtle than that. Some experiences, for example, may be the result of acting according to a conception at odds with that of the course – a phenomenon we observed in the course in operation. In such a case, the conception of the course *could* not coherently be modified simply to fit the experiences. What is required is a critical evaluation of the different conceptions at work behind the actions leading to the experiences in question, with the intention of understanding what subsequent action would best achieve the purposes of the course of study – and, naturally, acting upon that under-standing. At the very least, such deeper evaluation helps avoid merely *ad hoc* and often contradictory changes to a course which can have a destructively fragmenting effect, for both staff and students.

Action in the light of evaluation: student responses to learning packages

Student responses to learning packages were dealt with by individual facilitators or by the teaching team where appropriate. An example of how the running of a learning package changed in the light of student responses may be illustrated in regard to the second learning package students undertook in Year 1. In response to the question 'What in your view are the worst features of the learning package?' many students had commented on the repetitiveness of some material and on the lack of new material in the second block of the package (verbatim student responses are given in Appendix 8).

As a result of teaching-team evaluation of these responses, two modifications were made to the learning package. First, the duration of the package was reduced from two weeks to a week and a half. Second, members of the teaching team returned to the clinical records used as source data for the design of the original package, and extracted more data for use in Block 2 of the package. Responses to the modified package from students in the succeeding year indicated that these changes had improved the package.

Systematic co-ordination of the design and review of packages across each semester, each year and across the course as a whole enabled such adjustments to be accommodated constructively. With such co-ordination, a reduction of half a week in the duration of one package could be absorbed in additional time in other activity where it was needed during the semester. Importantly, it also meant that adjustments could be made without loss to the coherency of the course, and that an accumulation of adjustments would not allow 'incremental creep' to produce unnoticed imbalances in student workload over the course, 'bottlenecking' of due dates for assessment items and so on.

Action in the light of evaluation: open forums

As described earlier, forums gave students an opportunity to raise and discuss particular issues. An example is given in Figure 9.4, showing student comments on one of the issues they raised, namely, assessment. The comment '8 groups negative' and '1 group even' indicates that of the nine small groups into which the forum was divided to discuss the issue, eight groups considered the negative items more significant than the positive items, and one group considered them about even.

The weight of negative responses in this case is a good example of an issue causing considerable concern to students, and an evaluation process which gathered information on the issue in preparation for appropriate action to be taken. It also illustrates two further matters. First, it illustrates the need for staff development on the important issue of assessment in any course whether problem-based or not. Second, it illustrates how inadequately prepared course materials and questionable practices can undermine a course. Overcoming these difficulties would clearly require detailed attention and, in the case of inadequate understanding of the course, could be expected to be a longer-term process. However, immediate steps could also be taken in response to legitimate student concerns. Action in regard to the comment 'Inconsistency in marking' provides a useful example.

Five steps were taken to overcome what is clearly a legitimate ground for concern. First, facilitators agreed among themselves to undertake informal marking moderation through discussion of marking standards and practices with each other. Second, marking across groups was undertaken (i.e., facilitators marked assessment items from students in groups other than their own). Third, discussions of marking and marking results were undertaken during formal teaching-team meetings. Fourth, existing criteria given to students were specified in greater detail for the assessment categories 'well developed', 'developing' and 'unmet' (i.e., satisfactory standard not met). And, fifth, learning contracts were introduced so that students and staff could, within the established assessment criteria, negotiate the learning to be undertaken by students and how it was to be assessed.

The result of actions such as these taken in response to evaluation information may speak for itself. Students surveyed in the following year, near the end of Year 3, gave favourable views of their assessment. As we have seen in Figure

Positive	Negative	Changes
Learning package focus assists learning	Too broad	More report writing
	More time to re-submit – avoid overloading of re-submissions with due assignments	More weight to content rather than style
	Personal marking	More health based
		More anatomy & physiology
	Credentialling too loose	More nursing based
	Some groups failing all the time	
		Criteria more clearly written Discussion with group re: assessments before commencing
	Not enough information	
	Bias toward literature review	
	Lack of clarity of questions	Facilitators need to agree on criteria
	Inconsistency in marking	
	Extensions too easy	Not run concurrently with learning packages
	Too academically based	Finish learning package week before assignment due
	Last due dates too close to end of semester disadvantages country students	Random marking
	Writing to please facilitator	Just student number not name on assignments
	Question and marking criteria too vague	Need to be more related to health issues

	8 groups negative	1 group even

Figure 9.4: Example of an issue raised by students in an open forum assessment

9.1, student ratings for questions about 'Appropriate assessment' resulted in a score of forty-nine (on the scale −100 to 100), and this was in fact the highest score gained in any of the five scales (see also, for example, Appendix 10 which includes the item 'Provided feedback through evaluation'. This item received the high mean score of student responses of 4.0 on a scale of 0–5, with 5 representing 'Very effective.')

Conclusion

Evaluation, then, is crucially important in the development of any problem-based learning course, a point appreciated by students as the following succinct and pertinent student comment illustrates:

> *Worth doing for future course development.*
>
> *Andrew, Year 3 student*

Evaluation is not a once in a while add-on activity extraneous to a course itself. This is not to deny the legitimacy and value of independent, occasional, external evaluations – but the latter are additional to, not a replacement for, integral, internal evaluation by participants. Moreover, evaluation as an integral part of a problem-based learning course has a role right from the beginning of planning. Proposals about the overall conception and detailed arrangements for a course need to be evaluated no less than does the later operation of the course in practice. When a course is running, evaluative information about various aspects of its operation can easily be side-lined and ignored unless effective processes have been established to engage this information with reflective discussion by staff on the course. These processes will be most effective when they are consistent with the nature and principles of problem-based learning itself – staff themselves need to model processes of identifying situations in need of improvement, of generating ideas to gain any desired improvement, of evaluating knowledge and information relevant to this task, of working co-operatively in seeking the best solutions, and the like. As a staff development activity this serves not only to allow the sharing of experience and knowledge of various practices in operation with others, and thus for staff to develop their own teaching practices as part of improving the course, but also to help new staff to find their way in a new situation. Not least, rigorous evaluation in these various ways can help show that well-designed and run problem-based learning courses have nothing to fear from scrutiny.

Chapter 10
Beginning from where you are

Don Margetson, Marie Cooke and Michele Don

Beginning from where you are is an important principle in problem-based learning. It is a rather obvious principle, but many forms of learning do not recognise it as fully in practice as does problem-based learning. As we suggested in the previous chapter, one possible future line of development is for problem-based learning to be introduced in parts of courses of study, perhaps with a view to building on that modest beginning to more comprehensive problem-based practice. This is an attractive prospect. Few teachers in higher education can look forward to the possibility of designing and developing a whole degree programme from scratch. For many, the example of a fully problem-based learning degree course in a new school of nursing which we described in earlier chapters may appear to be of marginal relevance to their established contexts of long-standing practice. In this chapter we will, therefore, look at how teachers in existing non-problem-based courses might move towards the practice of problem-based learning in whatever educational contexts they currently find themselves.

In exploring this issue we will take the opportunity to reflect upon and remind ourselves of matters discussed in earlier chapters, including the introduction where we considered some philosophical implications of problem-based learning. This will enable us to summarise and draw attention to some important points for those adopting problem-based learning, whether in whole or in part. We therefore see the question of a limited adoption of some aspects of problem-based learning in a positive light. It is not a matter of being stuck with second-best; rather, it is a matter of beginning from where you are and working constructively from that realistic position towards the benefits deriving from problem-based learning. Let us approach the question by sketching a typical scenario which many university teachers will have experienced in some form or another on many campuses in different parts of the world.

So what about the tutorial after the lecture?

Imagine two colleagues walking across campus. As they walk to their offices – Chang's in the nursing building, Liz's in the science building – they are discussing the degree course on which they both teach. Chang has just taken a tutorial on the special nursing required by people being treated with certain drugs, and is complaining that his students don't seem to have a clue about the biochemical effects of drugs on the behaviour of human beings and that this makes it exasperatingly difficult to convey to students how important the special nursing care is. Liz isn't too happy herself about the students, for she finds them frustratingly uninterested in her lectures on just that topic – they are always complaining, she says, about the irrelevance of all the minutiae of complicated biochemical explanations. Their parting joke to each other is how interesting it might be to put on a kind of Punch and Judy show in which he pops up saying, 'Look, this is what happens to your sense of balance when you're on drug X', and she pops up saying, 'Yes, and this is why your sense of balance deserts you when you've taken drug X', etc.

But of course they know that there is no chance of that happening, given that nursing is nursing and science is science; that their respective academic departments are, in the current straitened circumstances in which universities find themselves working, hard-pressed just to support their own disciplines without having to collaborate with others; and so on. Nonetheless, Liz and Chang feel deeply that something can be done to help students learn more effectively. What could I do, they each ask themselves as they take the paths to their separate buildings: couldn't I perhaps modify my tutorials in some constructive way, even if – jokes about Punch and Judy shows aside – serious co-operative teaching across departments is too ambitious initially?

An example of one small step in a practice which could, with development, evolve towards the kind of fully problem-based learning we have described in the earlier part of this book is the following. Imagine that, as it happens, during the week following her walk with Chang, Liz comes across an article which describes how a traditional subject in a degree course was transformed into problem-based learning mode. The article, 'The introduction of a problem-based option into a conventional engineering degree course' (Cawley 1989), includes a description of the structure of tutorials which sparks an idea in Liz's mind. What if, instead of simply giving students exercises in tutorials on biochemical reactions and processes, she gets them to simulate a situation in which it would be important to communicate the biochemical causes of the effects of certain drugs?

Suppose, she thinks, I divide the tutorial group into two smaller groups, each of which is given the role of a technical authoring group in a drug-research company with the task of writing a clear explanation for practising nurses of the effects of drug X on those taking them, and the biochemical reasons for those effects? Instead of each student individually doing exercises in preparation for the next tutorial, they will, in the two small groups, write the required professional document. At the subsequent tutorial, the two small groups will exchange documents and the tutorial will compare and discuss them, with Liz helping students to ensure that the scientific knowledge put forward is accurate.

This is, of course, far from a fully problem-based approach, since students still go to regular lectures, the tutorials follow the lectures and the tutorials are still largely thought of as testing student understanding of the material presented in lectures. On the other hand, what happens in the tutorial is markedly different from the traditional practice. In the traditional tutorial they might be given an exercise along the lines of 'Explain what would happen if enzyme z were introduced into the digestive tract in the presence of drug X'. That is simply an exercise in biochemistry. In contrast, in the tutorial as modified by Liz, students at first glance seem to be doing something belonging to a communications course in the arts faculty rather than a biochemical exercise in the science faculty. But it is, of course, not a case simply of *either* one thing *or* the other thing – what students are learning to communicate is an explanation of a biochemical process. To do this satisfactorily they will certainly need to understand the biochemical process. In addition, the importance of understanding the biochemical process becomes clear through having to relate this to a further purpose. This gives some expression to problem-based learning principles, such as actively relating one aspect of knowledge to others, integrating the use of knowledge in contexts of use, and working co-operatively with others. In bald terms, Liz's modified tutorial looks less like a pure information-acquisition session and more like a problem-based learning session designed to result in effective learning.

Is it problem-based learning?

But in what way is this a problem-based learning approach rather than any other kind of approach to teaching and learning? Let us consider six crucial aspects which together make up problem-based learning. This will help us to do two things. First, it will summarise crucial aspects of the material in earlier chapters and thereby provide part of a usefully brief means of evaluating the extent to which a given educational practice is a case of problem-based learning. Second, it will enable us to consider how some characteristics of problem-based learning can be introduced in conventional teaching courses in a small way at first, with possible further development as interest and opportunity arise. The six characteristics are: (1) problem-focus from the beginning; (2) initial enquiry; (3) consulting resources; (4) reflection, refinement, development; (5) iterations of 1–5; (6) conclusion. In brief outline, each of these can be described in the following way.

(1) *Problem-focus from the beginning*

A particular teaching session (e.g., a problem-based tutorial) begins with a problematic situation relevant to the area of study. The situation is put forward in an appropriate way (in the case of health-care professions this could be a video of an incident; a simulated patient; written description of a presenting client and some symptoms; documents about a public health matter (e.g., a government health report, a memo from a director of nursing to agency staff). It is important not to be misled by the phrase 'the problem' in such situations. What is commonly referred to as 'the problem' is short-hand for a cluster of related problems in a context. 'The problem' is the focal problem – the main, or primary, question on which attention is concentrated. No problem can be understood in pure isolation, so other matters are always implied. The phrase 'the problem' is useful as a brief way of referring to a complex phenomenon.

(2) *Initial enquiry*

Active enquiry into the problem-situation is then conducted – e.g., identifying clearly what seems to be the problem, tentatively identifying possible explanations of its occurrence, clarifying what learning is needed in order to understand the problem better and determine whether the possible explanations stand up to more informed scrutiny, organising how this knowledge and information will be gathered and brought to bear, etc.

(3) *Consulting resources*

Relevant resources are consulted – textbooks, journal articles, laboratory work, teachers or other persons where appropriate, and so on, for the purpose of the student's learning what needs to be learned, as identified during the initial enquiry.

(4) *Reflection, refinement, development*

The learning resulting from the study of the selected resources is brought to bear on the problem as initially understood, and the implications of those results for the initial formulation of the problem are worked out. Accordingly, understanding of the problem may be modified and refined; further inquiry develops this understanding and determines which explanations are worth pursuing, which can be dropped, and whether new ones are necessary.

(5) *Iterations of 1–5*

The process is repeated as required. The level of detail and depth to which learning can proceed in regard to this problem-situation will be dependent, among other things, on the time available. There is no simple 'right' amount of time.

(6) *Conclusion*

The conclusion to the learning process will depend on the area of study under consideration. In nursing, for example, an appropriate conclusion would be a diagnosis of the problem-situation (that is, the situation in need of improvement), a plan of action to deal with it and a specified means of evaluating whether the plan of action was successful, to what extent, and how it might have been improved. This may or may not form part of the formal assessment of learning by the student which would, as in any course of study, have to be assessed at some time.

It is important to draw attention to some implications of this outline. First, the characteristics outlined above indicate that in principle problem-based learning is not restricted to any particular area of study, or even to broad areas such as professional studies. It can operate in any area of study. Second, while group work adds extremely valuable qualities to the student learning experience, as earlier chapters have shown, it is not strictly a necessary part of problem-based learning. An individual in isolation could follow the process outlined above. Indeed, in principle this is not unlike the process a research student would undertake – a point which suggests that problem-based learning is a way to breaking down artificial barriers between undergraduate and postgraduate study and, in particular, between teaching and research in university work (Margetson 1993). However, given the very great advantages group work brings, it would be extremely unwise not to use it wherever possible in a course of study. Third, not all forms of teaching which make use of problems in some way are appropriately described as teaching in a problem-based learning way.

The third point is well illustrated by the example – not invented, but based on an actual exchange – of the person who refers to problems in their teaching and therefore concludes that what they are doing is problem-based learning. Asked to explain this, the person (Jo, let us say) responded along the following lines: 'I give three lectures a week, run a three-hour lab in which students do experiments related to the lectures, and have a one-hour tutorial in which students solve problems taken from the textbook. The tutorial problems test their understanding of the lecture material; that material is necessary to their solving the problems, so my subject is an example of problem-based learning.' Faced with this kind of view of what problem-based learning is, confusion tends to reign, since, on such a view, practically anything can be described as problem-based learning. This risk is especially severe in potentially transitional situations – such as the one in which Liz and Chang find themselves – since those are just the situations in which 'problems' in some sense or other already exist but in which any more developed view and practice of problem-based learning is not yet present. Reference to the six characteristics given above shows that virtually the only resemblance between Jo's case and problem-based learning is that the term 'problem' occurs in both.

Much of what teachers and learners currently do is related to problems, even if only implicitly. A move towards problem-based learning is not, therefore, quite such a large step as at first appears to be the case. Teachers could reflect on what they currently teach, on their current course structures and on their teaching practices and find in this great potential for giving fuller acknowledgement to the place of problems in education. But if there is, as it were, so much problematic potential just below the surface, why does it appear to be so difficult to move towards problem-based teaching?

The traditional approach to education has been founded largely on a view that knowledge is a foundation and must be transmitted by the teacher to the learner before anything else can take place. As there is a vast amount of knowledge – itself growing exponentially – the focus has been very heavily on a view of teaching as the transmission of foundational knowledge. To a large extent, 'problems' have been seen as a peripheral element in this, at best treated as simple, atomistic entities to be dealt with as brief exercises in tutorials. At worst they have been seen not to be part of formal education at all, but left for graduates to encounter and cope with in the 'real' world as best they can after they have left the ivory tower. This kind of conception has systematically obscured the centrality of problems in the development of knowledge and understanding and, consequently, has missed the significance of problems in education (Margetson 1994). Development towards problem-based learning, whether fully or in part, does therefore require serious reconsideration of deep-seated assumptions about knowledge, understanding, teaching and learning.

A traditional pattern of lectures plus laboratory plus tutorial (in which brief, quite artificial, problems are solved) reflects the six characteristics outlined above hardly at all. Compared with an example of problem-based learning such as described in the earlier chapters of this book, the six characteristics are either virtually invisible apart from the explicit use of the word 'problem', or contradicted (as in the first characteristic, since students do not begin with a problem but with lectures in which knowledge is transmitted). This leads to two questions which we will now address: why are these characteristics of problem-based learning important; and can they be used in existing courses without converting a whole curriculum to problem-based learning?

Why these characteristics of problem-based learning are important

As we have noted earlier, in a review of the research literature Biggs (1989:17) describes four conditions which facilitate effective learning, namely: a well-structured knowledge base; learner activity; interaction with others; and a context of motivation. Gibbs (1992), we also noted, in an account of various innovations in higher education, drew attention to the fact that problem-based learning satisfies all four conditions. This provides strong support for the educational benefit of fully problem-based learning. In addition, the four conditions provide a further means of clarifying what it would mean to introduce aspects of problem-based learning into current educational practices. By way of example, consider some aspects of the first two characteristics in regard to two cases, A and B.

In A, the teacher appears at first glance to exemplify the first characteristic of problem-based learning by beginning with a problem-situation, which the teacher carefully describes in class. The second characteristic also appears to be satisfied, since the teacher pursues an initial enquiry in class, outlining some explanations of the occurrence of the problem, identifying what further knowledge would be required in order to deal with it, and so on. In B, on the other hand, the teacher satisfies the same two characteristics by showing students in class a video clip of a problem-situation, into which students then begin an initial enquiry, clarifying what the problem is, outlining possible explanations and so on.

Clearly, A and B contrast sharply on two, and possibly three, of Biggs's four conditions. In A, there is little if any learner activity and no interaction between learners; in B, learner activity and interaction between learners is an integral part of the process of learning, facilitated by the teacher. In addition, and partly in virtue of these two conditions themselves, B is likely to provide a more motivating context of learning than A. On the fourth condition – a well-structured knowledge base – A and B may be similar, although the way in which this base was present would differ significantly. That is, in A, the teacher would be *presenting* a well-structured knowledge base; in B the teacher would be *facilitating student learning* of a well-structured knowledge base – in two ways.

First, the questions the teacher asked, and (where appropriate) the suggestions and the challenges made to students, would be informed by the knowledge base. Questioning, for example, while sometimes being appropriately general ('Why do you think that?') would in other cases be quite knowledge-specific ('Are there any reasons to think that amphetamines would be effective in counteracting excess levels of enzyme z in the lower intestinal tract?', a question which teachers, in virtue of their knowledge, would be in a position to ask at an appropriate time). Second, since a course of study in a professional area would be preparing students to satisfy quite detailed and comprehensive knowledge requirements, the set of problems on which they worked during their course would be selected to ensure that they gained the required knowledge in the professional area. In this sense, the set of problems is selected and organised so that student learning of a well-structured knowledge base will be facilitated. The importance of the careful design of a *whole course of study* (such as an entire degree programme), within which individual problem-situations are located and sequenced, cannot be over-emphasised.

If we considered Jo's example again in terms of this combination of the six problem-based learning characteristics and Biggs's four conditions, it becomes clear that Jo's teaching falls a long way short of problem-based learning. Indeed, if Jo took a very information-transmission view of lectures, reserving the tutorials as the occasion on which problems would be presented and dealt with, then Jo's teaching would fall short even of case A that we have just outlined. With this in mind let us turn to the question of whether existing teaching and learning situations can make use of the characteristics in part.

Is adaptation in existing courses possible?

An answer to this question grows out of the previous discussion. In terms of the six problem-based learning characteristics and Biggs's four conditions, case B was clearly problem-based; case A and Jo's example were not – although, as we have noted, there were elements even in those two cases which are related to problem-based learning. Suppose that Jo is in fact a colleague in Liz's faculty, and that it was Jo who had been explaining to Liz how her course was problem-based. However, having been persuaded that her course was not really problem-based at all, and being sympathetic to the idea of problem-based learning, Jo and Liz explore how they might adapt some of their teaching.

They like Liz's idea of a tutorial where students work in groups on the problem of a technical authoring group in a drug-research company with the task of writing a clear explanation for practising nurses of the effects of drug X on those taking them, and of the biochemical reasons for those effects. Through discussion of it, they refine the idea. Questions of whether the proposal is possible in one tutorial session arise. They develop the idea in such a way that in one version a very simple drug is involved, the explanation of which might be appropriate for a single tutorial session. In a second, more realistic, version, a complex drug is involved which would require student work over a number of weeks. In this version, the subject-content that would previously have been dealt with over the same number of weeks is incorporated; that is, in tackling the problem and preparing their documents, students would learn this subject-content. A further development Liz and Jo introduce is that, instead of tutorial sub-groups simply exchanging documents, Jo and Liz agree that it would be better for a group to present their account verbally to the others, and then to exchange documents to compare and discuss them in greater detail. This will, they feel, help students to learn how to convey important scientific ideas clearly in a spoken form, as well as presenting them in a written form more open to detailed evaluation for scientific adequacy, communicative effectiveness and so on.

This kind of adaptation within an existing course clearly satisfies some essential characteristics of problem-based learning. The students begin with a problem and proceed directly to active enquiry; there is thus learner activity and inter-action between learners. The problem they are working on simulates an actual complex situation in which scientific knowledge needs to be understood and used effectively, and the problem-situation presented to students has been carefully designed so that students will need to gain the relevant knowledge in the course of tackling the problem – thereby ensuring that they learn not only the necessary subject-content but also how to inquire effectively, how to co-operate well with others and how to bring closely related matters together in a coherent way.

Equally clearly, this is a limited adaptation in the existing course. Lectures remain central, and the tutorial comprises perhaps only 10 per cent of the contact time in the course. However, as experience and confidence in this kind of problem-based structure and facilitative teaching within it increased, further development might be contemplated. A next step might, for example, be to move from a 3:1 lectures:tutorial arrangement to replacing one of the lectures with a problem-based tutorial along the lines just described. If timetabling allowed this, the previous lecture and tutorial periods might be brought together, providing a valuable two-hour tutorial opportunity rather than the more usual one-hour.

Many other possibilities will be available in different contexts and situations. In our hypothetical scenario, at some stage Liz and Jo may take up the original suggestion made by Chang and Liz that they share joint tutorials, thus beginning a cross-departmental co-operative arrangement which would increase the inter-disciplinary nature of teaching sessions with potentially significant benefit to students. In general, it would be important to review this kind of piecemeal expansion of problem-based learning after some experience had been gained. Further piecemeal expansion might be less economical than putting planning and design energies into redesigning larger segments – or even a whole course of study. This possibility takes development beyond the realm of the individual to a more systematic institutional involvement in educational development.

Institutional effects and the isolated academic

While valuable modifications of a problem-based kind can, then, be introduced by individuals into the subject they teach without direct implications for other parts of a whole course of study, there may come a point when more systematic institutional involvement becomes essential to further development. What could, for example, Jo, Liz and Chang do in this situation? An important factor would be to involve senior members of a department in considering the benefits of extending problem-based learning approaches within each department and possibly in inter-departmental co-operation. This possibility does, however, depend on local conditions. It would be most likely to succeed where senior members of a department were sympathetic and open to such development. Where indifference, or hostility – or, perhaps worst of all, mere lip-service support not backed up by a genuine willingness to take the matter up seriously – were found, the road to development would be longer and harder. In this case, individuals or groups might have to concentrate largely on their own areas, and work away patiently at seeking development in other areas of the courses they were involved in. Each situation would have to be dealt with on its own merits and potential for development.

In any case, a factor such as the involvement of senior members of a department needs to be combined with other significant factors in the success of educational innovation such as the introduction of problem-based learning. A good example of a list of such factors, some of which we have mentioned in earlier chapters, is found in Figure 10.1.

Adopting the advice given in this list can lead to significant overall institutional benefits. Not least among these is the contribution these factors can make to developing a 'learning organisation' (Senge 1990), a notion implying that the organisation has the capacity not only to satisfy quite obvious functions (teaching students, say) in a minimal way, but also to improve its performance. The learning organisation facilitates creativity among its members so that its purposes are achieved more richly and meaningfully than is possible when merely satisfying minimal immediate needs is regarded as satisfactory. The idea of the learning organisation sounds remarkably like the idea of what a university should be like.

Does it, then, have any connection with the kind of scenario we sketched involving Chang, Jo and Liz as a hypothetical example of the kind of situation facing many in actual educational contexts? That scenario – which follows some of the advice in the list given by Boud and Feletti – implies a much more developed context of discussion, dialogue and co-operation than is often found in regard to teaching and learning in higher education institutions. These vital academic qualities are among just those which characterise a learning organisation. They are sometimes lost sight of under the pressures of rapidly expanding higher education systems

a clear purpose and philosophy outlined to students and faculty

acquisition of sufficient resources: funds, teachers, equipment, clerical and educational support, teaching space

dean's support or leadership

nominal support (at least) from departmental heads

faculty genuinely committed to its trial and further improvement

students willing to accept greater responsibility for their learning

a curriculum committee with clear communication to faculty

a suitable project leader with acceptable autonomy to proceed

an explicit commitment to specific project deadlines

facilities for appropriate staff–student contact and self-directed studies

plans for the recognition of teaching effort and excellence (rewards not just for research achievements)

regular planning and review meetings involving faculty, support staff and students

adequate support networks and encouragement for both faculty and students

opportunities for faculty to reflect, expound, benefit from their experiences with the approach

political support for innovators when facing faculty 'resistance'

observation of problem-based learning in action, access to consultants

Figure 10.1: Checklist of elements – getting problem-based learning started
Source: Boud and Feletti 1991: 56

required to function with reduced support per student. Yet it is just qualities such as these which are crucial in enabling organisations such as universities to identify, understand and respond in a responsible way to the needs – both perceived and as yet unrecognised – of the communities of which they are part.

None the less, as we have seen, individuals can take some initiatives in improving educational practice despite the questionable policies of governments and overly compliant institutional managements. Such initiatives can generate precisely the kind of context which fosters the learning that comes from a rigorously problem-based educational practice – and not only for the individuals concerned but also for the organisation of which they are part. In the remainder of this chapter we will outline further possible ways in which individuals and groups of individuals in co-operation can introduce practices of a proto-problem-based learning kind which could help improve the quality of learning and teaching in higher education.

Facilitation

Whether the initial change to problem-based learning is instigated in a minimal way or more broadly will depend on the particular situation – the Boud and Feletti checklist outlined in Figure 10.1 and the discussion of the six crucial characteristics of problem-based learning described in this chapter may help you assess where and to what extent change is possible. However, as the transition to problem-based learning becomes more evident you will also need to focus on the move from the more traditional role of teaching to facilitating students' enquiry and critical thinking. Once you have the teaching material, structured around real problem-situations, which incorporate the concepts you wish to address in a tutorial, laboratory or course, ways of encouraging students to engage with the material creatively and critically need to be considered. Chapter 7 details how staff can be helped to understand and feel more comfortable with the facilitative role as outlined in Chapter 3. From our experience, the most useful means of gaining this understanding is through participating in a tutorial facilitated by an experienced teacher. Some of you may not have access to such people and will need to think more broadly about possibilities for using such a resource. For example, you may combine reading about the facilitative role with exchanging thoughts, ideas, comments, etc., with an experienced facilitator over the telephone. It may be possible for you to organise with an experienced facilitator to video-tape, audio-tape or transcribe a problem-based tutorial for viewing, listening to or reading. This could also be combined with a debriefing session over the telephone to allow comments, reflections or questions that may arise for you to be answered. An alternative strategy may be for you to video-tape a session with you facilitating colleagues in working through the problem-situation which you have designed and written. This tape could then be forwarded to an experienced person for review and comment. This gives the added advantage of gaining some sense of how the problem-situation works in terms of triggering the issues identified as needing to be addressed in your subject or module.

Timetabling and resources

Other issues that may be raised in discussing the changes with colleagues are the extra time and resources needed for student learning. Both of these issues need to be addressed with some flexibility and creativity: firstly, the question of extra time needed for student learning. In the long term, fewer contact sessions between staff and students are necessary within the problem-based learning situation and this, combined with some flexible timetabling, can address this issue successfully. The usual contact hours per week for students for a course may remain the same; some of this may, however, be allocated to self-directed learning. If usual contact hours are five, then maybe two hours of this is set aside for tutorial time and three hours allocated to self-directed learning where students gain access to various resources to assist the achievement of the learning goals identified in the problem-based tutorial – Chapter 1 outlines in detail the ways in which students can be facilitated to identify their learning needs.

Secondly, with the issue of resourcing, there should not be a need for extra resources, except for some information about problem-based learning for students. Written texts, videos, etc., that are available for the tutorial, laboratory or course will still be appropriate and relevant. Resources in terms of teaching space may need to be addressed. In facilitating small groups of students, more tutorial room space may be necessary; we have found, however, that there are creative ways in which difficulties can be overcome. For example, group rooms within libraries can be used; laboratories can be used by more than one small group concurrently; or any other teaching space which is available as well as outdoor areas may be used if appropriate. An alternative is to stagger student groups' meeting times so that less teaching space can be used over a longer period of time.

Converting a lecture-based course

As teachers become more comfortable and gain more confidence in the problem-based structure it may be possible to consider converting a totally lecture-based course within a degree. This will depend upon a range of variables as outlined in Figure 10.1, but may be encouraged if smaller-scaled problem-based work is evaluated by students and staff in terms of student learning outcomes.

The example which follows illustrates how a course entitled 'Evaluating Social Programs' could be converted from a traditional lecture-based course to a problem-based course. This subject has the following content areas: evaluation goals and objectives, social policy, social sciences, models of the state, implementing assessment, cost-effectiveness and cost-benefit analysis, and evaluation methods and research. This course runs over a fourteen-week semester with students allocated three hours of lecture time per week. In converting this course a number of 'real' social programmes could be structured as problem-situations to encourage students to enquire into, critically appraise, reflect upon and evaluate the concepts inherent in the content areas. The first 'real' problem-situation would address some of these concepts initially, with further problem-situations addressing them in more depth with the addition of more concept areas. Although Chapter 2 details in full how you might go about designing and writing learning material, the first block of learning material for the first problem-situation might be:

> **Block I**
>
> *In Queensland, drowning is responsible for more deaths in the 0–4 year age group than any other and 46.43 per cent of deaths by drowning can be attributed to the domestic pool (The Courier-Mail 24.3.90:2)*

> *The Child Accident Prevention Foundation of Australia (CAPFA) has identified four main contributing factors to swimming pool drownings. These are: 'Interruptions to supervision, Lack of adequate fencing, Poor maintenance of self-locking gates, Lack of adequate skill in resuscitation and emergency procedures' (1980:unnumbered page).*
>
> *You are the Director of Community Services. The Minister for Housing and Local Government has just announced in a press statement that a submission to Cabinet will be presented for state-wide legislation on the mandatory fencing of private swimming pools.*

The facilitator might encourage students to consider the material by introducing such questions as: Why is the government taking this action? Who are the possible winners and losers in regard to the policy? Who will implement the policy? What are the manifest and hidden goals and objectives of the policy? Are there any unintended consequences of the policy? and, What are the issues that may affect the evaluation of this policy?

The facilitator could assist the students to enquire actively into the situation considering the six aspects of problem-based learning outlined previously. This may take two hours of the second week's session. The first week's session would be used to orientate students to problem-based learning and the nature of the course of study. Students may then meet with the facilitator for one hour of the next two or three weeks' sessions to continue engaging with the problem. The remaining hours would be allocated to students' self-directed learning from their identified learning needs.

Conclusion

In this chapter we have addressed the task of introducing components of problem-based learning into established courses. Although the degree which we have outlined in previous chapters was designed and implemented as a fully integrated reiterative problem-based learning course, we see the adoption of sectional problem-based learning work as positive in terms of increasing the effectiveness of student learning.

What is essential in attempting to introduce problem-based learning into aspects of your teaching is to reflect on current teaching practices with a view to examining assumptions about knowledge, understanding, teaching and learning. As well, it is crucial to consider the factors which may help or hinder your ability to introduce aspects of problem-based learning to your tutorials, laboratories or courses and to work on what you can accomplish within local constraints. It may be that initially only small changes can be made to current teaching practices, but with positive evaluations from staff and students instigation of more changes may become possible. We have outlined some practical considerations and strategies which may assist in a successful transition of tutorials, laboratories and course to problem-based learning. If they work out – go bigger next year.

Good luck!

Chapter 11
What lessons – and where to?

Bob Ross

In the previous chapters of this book we have attempted to give you a sense of what is involved in a problem-based learning course, the major issues that arise and some guide to design, development, evaluation and implementation. In the process we hope we have conveyed some of our enthusiasm for the process and given an indication of the type of benefits students gain from such an approach. In this chapter we will review the earlier parts of the book briefly, and extract some general messages. We will outline the advances that we feel our experience brings to the field and make some comments about where problem-based learning might develop next. Finally, from our experience, we will give our views on the necessary conditions for mounting a successful problem-based course.

Beliefs about learning

I have learnt the art of learning. Something that will stay with me for the rest of my life.

Janet, Year 3 student

One of the most commonly stated views about higher education is that the most important thing we can achieve for our students is to help them to 'learn how to learn'. A number of the currently accepted beliefs about learning have been around for a considerable time. They include such beliefs as that people learn in different ways; people acquire knowledge and understanding by relating new ideas, circumstances and events to their existing knowledge and understanding; understanding is developed by applying existing knowledge to problems that are as close to real life as possible; learning is an active process; people learn from reflecting on their experience; one of the best ways to learn something is to teach it to others; understanding is developed by exploring ideas with other students; and people need to be able to try their skills and understanding in a safe, non-threatening environment. In addition, it has been recognised for a considerable time that teachers should see themselves as facilitators of learning as well as knowledgeable experts in their field.

It is our contention that the type of course that we have outlined in this book meets all these beliefs to an extent not found in any other approach to higher education.

If you recall Chapter 1 you will identify activities illustrated there that relate to each of these beliefs. Most of them are further emphasised in the subsequent chapters. We will take each of the above ideas and give an example to illustrate our contention.

People learn in different ways

Like a number of the beliefs this is almost a truism, and all students will, of course, learn in their own ways. However, very few courses make any attempt to accommodate the different ways in which students learn. The advice in Chapter 2 to incorporate as wide a range of approaches as available when developing trigger material for learning packages is, in part, an explicit attempt to meet these variations. Similar advice occurred in Chapter 4 where it was seen that a range of approaches has been valuable in assisting students to integrate different areas of knowledge that are usually treated in isolation. In addition, the extent to which groups and individuals are given responsibility for developing their own strategies for defining their learning needs (see also Chapters 5, 6 and 8) is a further approach to accommodating these differences.

People acquire knowledge and understanding by relating new ideas, circumstances and events to their existing knowledge and understanding

As with the belief above, if this one has any validity then students will automatically have to do it for themselves. It is clear that they can be assisted in this task, and that such assistance enhances the learning experience. However, very few courses either take advantage of students' existing knowledge or make any attempt to assist this process. Most courses assume students have no knowledge at all, other than that 'covered' in the course itself. In the approach described in this book the initial session of each block is clearly designed to elicit students' existing knowledge of the topics to be explored. This base is then used to identify the group's learning needs for that block. By this process students have defined (and, incidentally, sharpened) their existing knowledge before they start to define their learning needs. Staff facilitate this process and use the information they gain in that process as one of the ways they define students' general learning needs.

Self-direction is the cornerstone of problem-based learning and this has helped me to build my confidence as I enter practice as an RN.
Charles, Year 3 student

I think the most powerful experience for me was when I finally came to terms with the fact that I was responsible for my own learning.
Mandy, Year 3 student

You will have seen that students are responsible for selecting the sources of information that they examine, and the ways that they examine them (Chapters 1, 2, 4, 5 and 9). Staff explicitly obtain guidance, directly from students, from observing their processes and from their questions, to contribute to the design of the fixed-resource sessions (see, for example, the descriptions in Chapters 3 and 6).

Understanding is developed by applying existing knowledge to problems that are as close to real life as possible

Each situation the students are asked to address is carefully selected and designed to be suitable for their level of development and as close to situations they will encounter in their professional practice as possible (see Chapter 2); as indicated in the previous section, each situation is approached in a way that assists students to clarify the knowledge that they already possess on each topic.

In my last placement my CNC [clinical nurse consultant] commented on my problem-solving abilities and how this had made me a good nurse. Many situations which may have been overwhelming to me were reduced as I used my problem-based learning techniques to solve them.
Tracey, Year 3 student

Learning is an active process

The process of the course explicitly involves a range of forms of 'active learning'. Throughout, it should be clear that students are very closely involved in learning activities designed by the team or developed themselves with the assistance of their facilitator (see Chapters 1, 2, 3 and 6).

People learn from reflecting on their experience

Throughout, students are encouraged to relate their previous experience to the issues they face. In addition, in some places in the course students are asked to keep a journal of their learning experiences, and are assisted to use their journal to reflect on those experiences. The course is designed so that they gain additional experience from the activities within the course itself and they are required to report their reflections on those experiences (see Chapters 1, 4, 5, 6 and 9).

One of the best ways to learn something is to teach it to others

Students are required to explain the information they have obtained for the group to their fellow group members and each group is required to explain to the other groups their results from, and responses to, the situations posed in selected blocks (see Chapters 2, 4, 8 and 9).

Understanding is developed by exploring ideas with other students

All of the group sessions, both those facilitated by staff and those entirely controlled by the students themselves, involve students in exposing their ideas and understandings with their colleagues (see Chapters 1, 2, 4, 5 and 9).

People need to be able to try their skills and understanding in a safe, non-threatening environment

The evolving development of the nursing laboratory experiences incorporates this requirement, as will laboratories in all nursing courses. As indicated in Chapter 5, and below, the advance in the course described here is the use of the laboratory to assist students to identify the social and communication skills nurses require in their practice, and to give them the opportunity to develop those skills in the laboratory.

Teachers should see themselves as facilitators of learning as well as knowledgeable experts in their field

Throughout it is clear that the staff role as facilitator is a vital feature of the process of any problem-based course (see Chapter 3). In our experience it is important to see the facilitator role as a continually evolving one, hence our emphasis in Chapter 8 on the need for ongoing discussions, analysis and reflection by the team. It is important that all members of the team see this activity as an integral part of the course, not an additional chore that can be let slip once the course is under way.

Our contribution to problem-based learning

Of course most of the features discussed above should occur in any problem-based course. Where the course described here breaks new ground is in the explicitly reiterative nature of the design and in the level of integration of all relevant areas of knowledge. So, for example, Chapter 4, detailing the ways in which relevant science knowledge was integrated, forms an important contribution to the field of problem-based learning. Our own development and understanding of the problems encountered, and successfully overcome, in this area would, by itself, have justified the project. But this was merely para''eled by the growth of our own understanding in all the areas outlined earlier.

For example, in a nursing course, the integration and incorporation into the process of learning of the clinical staff (see Chapters 6 and 7) was a major, and necessary, achievement – they became our collaborators in a way that none of us had experienced elsewhere, but, as Chapters 6 and 7 demonstrate, not without considerable commitment on our behalf, as well as on the part of our clinical colleagues.

Another contribution that our project made was in the area of the nursing laboratory. While this seems purely related to nursing, potentially it has much wider applications. As Chapter 5 demonstrated, the evolution of our use of the laboratory facility occurred as part of our problem-based process in action. It is not therefore surprising that the outcome was laboratory sessions entirely consistent with our problem-based approach. The process of evolution of the laboratory sessions is instructive in itself, but, in addition, the use of that type of facility to foster development of the non-psychomotor skills required in nursing practice is an innovation with much wider potential application. That type of integration is clearly much more achievable in a problem-based course than elsewhere, but could form a model for similar integration in many professional education courses.

Outcomes

Our whole project would have been interesting, but basically unsuccessful, if our graduates had not achieved the goals we set for them. (That these goals were appropriate for a degree in nursing was guaranteed by endorsement of the course by the relevant professional body.) While only a thorough evaluation of the performance of our graduates in their employment practice would supply a definitive demonstration of our success, we hope to have shown you throughout the book that our confidence is justified. In Chapter 2 we outlined one of the important guides we employed to ensure appropriate 'coverage' of both content and process: our concept matrix.

The type of evaluation that we suggest in the paragraph above would, incidentally, be a rare event for *any* university course, including the most traditional and well established.

What the book has demonstrated is the important role in this style of course of ongoing evaluation at all levels – not just at the level of the final outcomes (skills, knowledge, understanding, attitudes) demonstrated by the graduates. While evaluation should be a part of any academic course it has a vital, integrated role in the design and implementation of the type of course we have been discussing in this book (see Chapter 9).

The future?

How do we feel problem-based learning might develop from this point?

One obvious development for us, particularly as we are involved in a new school whose first students graduated at the end of 1993, is into the postgraduate arena. Our academic area is one in which there is a considerable demand for, and growth in, postgraduate coursework courses. It is an obvious development for us to use problem-based learning to meet this demand. We will have to be careful that we don't assume that all our postgraduate coursework students are familiar with a problem-based approach.

Many postgraduate coursework courses use some procedures similar to those used in problem-based learning (group work, project tasks, student responsibility for obtaining information, case-studies and the explicit use of students' experience). So some of the 'disorientation' experienced by students commencing problem-based learning courses might not be such an issue for postgraduate coursework students. However, not all our students will have had any of these experiences, even if they have undertaken some postgraduate coursework.

The extension of problem-based learning to postgraduate coursework courses would clearly be suitable for areas outside the health professions. As the development of courses at that level seems common at present in many fields the attractiveness of problem-based learning should grow. Indeed, it is likely that some faculties, departments and institutions might find problem-based learning an acceptable approach at postgraduate coursework level while reluctant to try it for their undergraduate course. This could, in time, see the spread downwards of the approach.

There are some academic areas where problem-based learning would seem to us to be ideal, but in which, as far as we are aware, there haven't been any projects. Teacher education seems a glaring case in point. Many sections of engineering education have embraced problem-solving methods in parts of their degrees, but we find it hard to understand why problem-based learning does not seem to have been taken up generally as a curriculum approach in engineering. It may be that the professional bodies are seen as an obstacle. But this would be in distinct contrast with our own experience, where even the international body has endorsed problem-based learning. Perhaps faculties of engineering have been reluctant to approach their professional bodies.

Problem-based learning has made considerable progress in areas of professional education but it would be our contention that there is no logical reason for it to be restricted to those areas. Indeed, the arguments at the start of this chapter would seem to apply equally to any area of university study. So we would be delighted to see humanities courses and those in 'pure' science experiment with the approach. Particularly in a period where science again seems to have lost its attractiveness to students, a new approach might revitalise that interest as well as help to ensure the relevance of science education to current social needs.

On a different level, the question of the feasibility of extending problem-based learning beyond on-campus full-time study has been posed to us. Particularly in the Australian context, we have frequently had the proposition put to us that problem-based learning could not be made accessible to off-campus students. We have, many years ago, heard similar claims about the inappropriate nature of distance education for a whole range of areas of study – science and technology being common – only to see such claims denied by successful distance education courses being developed in those fields. Our own approach is to be sceptical about any such 'it can't be done' claims until we have seen serious attempts to develop such courses. We take the same attitude to such claims about off-campus study and problem-based learning.

In other words, we will continue to believe that distance education courses based on a problem-based learning approach should be possible until we see serious attempts to develop such courses fail. From the emphasis in this book it is clear that one of the major hurdles to be faced by a distance education problem-based learning course would arise from our heavy reliance on student–student interaction and on the facilitation of group work as both a vital process in encouraging student learning and an important learning experience in itself. Without attempting, here, to undertake the initial design work for such a course, let us merely say that such an endeavour would certainly test the ingenuity of the design team, but that would be part of the excitement of being involved. One recent development that may well make such a project more feasible is the work that has been done over the last five or so years on computer-mediated communication as a learning tool.

Another similar extension of problem-based learning would be into the realm of continuing education. As with postgraduate coursework, courses in this area already share many common features with problem-based learning, so we see no reason why continuing education should not embrace problem-based learning as a very appropriate approach. In non-professional continuing education the motivation of the students would be likely to mean that the initial alienation that many full-time undergraduates experience with problem-based learning would be avoided.

Closer to our own area of study, we are convinced of the benefit problem-based learning can bring to client (patient) education. In our view one of the requirements for good practice in nursing is facilitating client empowerment. This was one of the basic goals of our course. You will have seen (in Chapter 5) some of the ways we assisted students to develop and practise the skills involved; instances occurred in other chapters, and some of the assessment items (see Chapter 8) explicitly addressed these concepts. We see a very obvious development from assisting our students to help their clients to the use of problem-based learning to assist clients directly to empower themselves.

Clearly the features of problem-based learning are ideal for this task: incorporating different knowledge backgrounds, experience and learning styles and assisting students to take responsibility for their own learning. Where we are dealing with an individual as a client we again meet the distance education issue of the extent to which problem-based learning relies on group interaction for its success. In this type of client education the secret may lie in seeing a different composition for learning groups. There seems no reason to restrict the group to fellow 'students', and considerable potential in exploring groups composed of friends, relatives and professional support workers. The same extension, necessary for the individual, would also have benefits for groups. We certainly see exciting possibilities in this area.

As far as problem-based learning itself is concerned, we would hope to see further development of the advances we feel that we have experienced in integration of all relevant areas of knowledge and in the design of reiterative courses. We also benefited considerably from the participation of health and other professionals, including our clinical facilitators, in the development of our course, and have detailed the advantages of this throughout the book. The one client group which we were less able to include in the initial development of the course was our own students. As the course was implemented, as we have explained, we gained considerable insights from students through the ongoing evaluation that is an integral part of our curriculum process. It would now be possible for us to incorporate student input into the design of packages in a more direct manner (as well as continuing the valuable existing evaluation procedures). This might well lead to further important developments in problem-based learning.

Conditions necessary for success

Throughout the book we have emphasised activities and features of the development of our own course that we felt were necessary to its success, so we will merely summarise our experience here.

Of prime importance is institutional support – expressed at the central level as well as vital at the faculty level and below. In Chapter 7 we emphasised the importance of obtaining the commitment of all the staff involved and outlined measures designed to ensure both that commitment and the necessary under-standing of the approach. For the circumstances where new staff are being appointed to participate in such a course, we emphasised some important issues that need to be addressed in appointment procedures. We discussed the role of professional bodies briefly above: their support can be very encouraging and their accreditation of the course vital.

Some of the support necessary for a successful problem-based learning course consists of recognition of the time required to develop the resources for such a course. An even more important issue is the manner in which the institution's reward structure deals with the rather different activities required to be recognised as teaching in a problem-based learning course.

The requirements for a completely new course, similar to our own experience, are slightly different from those required for the conversion of an existing course, although the important issues are identical. For a conversion the commitment of the team planning the change is again vital, but watching their colleagues in the process of designing and developing the course, and observing the impact on students, can act as a process for convincing some staff who don't wish to become involved, but are accommodated by 'seeing out' the old course while the new one is developed.

A common question that has been posed to us is whether it is possible to have part of a course designed on a problem-based approach (as distinct from the whole course being so designed). Our response is that there doesn't seem to be any particular reason why such a development should be impossible. However, some of the requirements for success would be considerably harder to meet. For example, institutional and faculty support would be more vital, if anything, and the support, or at least lack of opposition of colleagues teaching in other parts of the course would become important.

There may be some difficulties with timetabling student activities in a flexible enough manner to allow the time necessary for students to seek the information for their learning package, but this shouldn't be an impossible problem to resolve. Where problems are more likely to arise is from other staff complaining about the time students spend on their problem-based activities, instead of 'studying' other subjects. This complaint may have considerable validity, but is a pointed comment on the lack of activities designed in those other sections of the students' work.

In general we feel that sectional problem-based work is likely to encounter more difficulties than where the whole course is problem-based, and we have suggested some possible ways of introducing problem-based aspects of learning into more traditional programmes in Chapter 10.

One criticism of problem-based learning which can be translated into a requirement for success hinges on cost. This is generally a mythological dragon. The 'cost' of any course is the resources made available to it. The decline in resources for university teaching over the last twenty years is adequate illustration that staff are able to 'cut their coat according to the cloth'. There is, of course, a limit to the resource decreases that can be accommodated without damaging the quality of student learning. But we have seen no evidence that the limit differs for different curriculum approaches. Use of particular techniques and technologies may well have to be constrained – but that does not necessarily make a particular curriculum approach impossible or, indeed, less viable than others.

And technology?

We write this book in a period of considerable 'hype' about the ways new information technology is going to revolutionise education, and hence teaching. What impact will such developments have on problem-based learning?

As you will have realised from the material in this book (particularly Chapter 2), we have advised the use of a range of technological devices and technologies (by 'technologies' we mean the ways in which the devices are used). We envisage the whole gamut of approaches being employed: text, audio, video, computer-aided learning packages, simulations, role-play, question and answer sessions, spoken presentations, etc. One justification for the range of approaches is to cater for different students' preferences; a second is to accustom students to the full range of information sources they will meet later in life. Problem-based learning is a curriculum approach that does not rely on, or restrict use to, particular technological devices, or combinations thereof. We see no reason to believe that problem-based learning will stop being one of the most effective curriculum approaches to learning (and to learning to learn), if not *the* most effective approach, no matter what modern information technology offers university teachers and their students. The impact of information technology on university education will depend on the ingenuity of people – we anticipate that those committed to problem-based learning will prove no less ingenious than any others, and probably more so. We ourselves are convinced that some of the new interactive multimedia technologies hold great promise for additional resources for problem-based learning courses; student work, in groups, on such 'packages' has real potential to assist understanding as well as to hone group interaction skills.

And us?

We have been involved in an exciting and rewarding experience as we developed the course that prompted this book. We have tried to share our experience with you and hope that we have also conveyed our excitement. As the quotations that we have shared with you amply demonstrate, our students also had a rewarding learning experience. May you and yours have the same.

Appendices

Appendix 1: Processing framework

A. *Problem-based tutorial*

Some crucial questions	Some useful prompts
1. Is there a situation in need of improvement?	• analyse the data • identify cues*
2. What is/are the situation(s) in need of improvement?	• write down this/these situations
3. What are your possible explanations for these situations?	• list tentative hypotheses • which are the most likely hypotheses?
4. What do you need to know in order to confirm or reject these explanations?	• list learning needs
5. Where might you find what you need to know?	• identify possible resources • library videos, persons, experience, etc.
6. How will you best organise yourselves to discover what you need to know?	• determine resources to be pursued • plan your group's activities for self-directed study • decide how you will share this information with your group

B. Self-directed study (3–6 hours)

C. Situation review tutorial

Some crucial questions	Some useful prompts
1. How does the knowledge you have gained help you to confirm, hold or reject your hypotheses?	• share information • review hypotheses in the light of information
2. Do you have need for further information?	• list the questions that the group have answered in fixed resource sessions

D. Situation summary tutorial

Some crucial questions	Some useful prompts
1. Will the knowledge you have gained enable you to accept, reject or hold hypotheses in order to make clinical judgements?	• review SINI • review hypotheses
2. What clinical judgements can you make in light of confirmed, rejected or held hypotheses?	• with further information, review SINIs • review hypotheses
3. What is the best way of acting on your clinical judgements?	Develop an action plan: • identify goals • identify ways to achieve goals • identify ways of reviewing your plan

E. Review of learning packages

Some crucial questions	Some useful prompts
1. What do you think you have learned by working through this package?	• how might this help you in your work as a nurse? • what are your reflections on the group process during this LP? • record your reflections in your journal

Year 1		Semester 1										Semester 2					
Health		LP 1	LP 2	LP 3	LP 4	LP 5	LP 6	LP 7	LP 8	LP 9	LP 10	LP 1	LP 2	LP 3	LP 4	LP 5	LP 6
Knowledge	Sexuality		X	X			X	X			X		X				
	Aging									X	X						
	Self-care		X	X	X		X	X			X	X	X				
	Family adaptation		X				X	X		X	X		X				
	Dependence/independence		X	X	X	X	X	X				X	X		X		
	Migrant health					X							X				
	Health		X	X	X	X	X	X	X	X	X	X	X	X		X	
	Wellness		X	X	X	X	X	X	X	X	X	X	X	X		X	
	Epidemiology		X	X	X	X	X			X	X	X	X	X		X	X
	Diagnostic investigations		X									X		X		X	X
	Complications HIV infection																X
	Pathology										X						X
	Health breakdown		X				X				X	X		X	X	X	

Skills													
Assessment of health	X		X	X	X	X	X	X	X	X			X
Preparation for death													X
Communication with dying													X
Individual & family support		X		X	X	X		X	X	X		X	
Mental health assessment								X		X			
Preparation for surgery								X		X			
Post-operative care								X		X			
Family assessment		X	X	X	X		X	X	X	X	X		X
Infant assessment											X	X	X

Attitudes													
Inquiry – processing	X	X	X	X	X	X	X	X	X	X	X	X	X
Data collection	X	X	X	X	X	X	X	X	X	X	X	X	X
Social and political	X	X	X	X	X	X	X	X	X	X	X	X	X
Non-judgemental respect	X	X	X	X									X
Human rights	X	X	X	X									X
Choice	X	X	X										X
Dying													X
Homosexuality													X
Stereotyping	X	X		X								X	X
Stigma	X	X		X		X						X	X
Effects of hospitalisation											X		
Beliefs and values	X	X	X	X	X	X	X	X	X	X	X	X	X
Aging as wellness	X	X	X	X	X		X	X	X	X	X	X	X
Responsibility self-care	X	X	X	X	X	X	X	X	X	X	X	X	X
Cultural awareness		X	X										

Appendix 3: Dialysis experiment

1. When you enter the lab divide into groups around each of the benches where equipment is provided for you to perform the experiment to accompany this worksheet.

2. This is a simple experiment to explore the principles of dialysis as they apply to both peritoneal dialysis and haemodialysis. You have 4 dialysis bags (dialysis tubing knotted at each end) and 4 beakers labelled 1–4. These contain respectively:

Tubing	Beaker
1 starch solution	1 iodine solution
2 iodine solution	2 starch solution
3 starch + iodine	3 water
4 copper sulphate solution	4 water

NB starch + iodine react together irreversibly to give a blue compound. Check this for yourselves by taking a small amount of the starch solution from beaker 2 and adding a few drops of iodine from beaker 1.

3. Make notes of

   - size/firmness or turgor of the bags
   - colour of all the solutions
   - are the bags 'water tight'? (How can you check?)

4. Place each of the dialysis bags into the beaker of the same number ie 1–1, 2–2, etc.

Set the beakers to one side while you work through the following worksheet. Leave them for at least 20–30 minutes before looking at them again.

Worksheet

1. An understanding of the following science terms/concepts will enhance your learning about dialysis:
   - osmosis
   - diffusion
   - active transport
   - passive transport
   - molecular weight
   - filtration
   - dialysis
   - dialysate

- osmolarity/osmolality
- concentration
- semi-permeable membrane
- hypertonic/hypotonic/normotonic

- metabolic acidosis
- asepsis
- gravity

Explain how these terms relate to an explanation of peritoneal dialysis or haemodialysis.

2. What are the differences between haemodialysis and peritoneal dialysis?

3. Compare the advantages and disadvantages of both systems of dialysis.

Return to thinking about the current experiment.

4. What do you predict will have happened in each beaker in the time since you added the dialysis bags?

Make observations of the beakers and dialysis bags, noting

– any colour changes
– any colour movement
– the size/firmness or turgor of the bags.

5. How do these changes compare to your predictions?

6. What comparisons can you draw between this experiment and peritoneal dialysis?

7. What comment can you make about the molecular weight (size) of the compounds either originally in the dialysis bags or in the beakers? (The dialysis membrane used has a mol. wt. exclusion of 12,000.)

8. What conclusions can you draw about the movement of substances across the dialysis membrane?

9. Use these conclusions – principles – to expand on your understanding of what occurs during peritoneal dialysis and haemodialysis.

10. Can dialysis be used to *totally* remove a waste product such as urea from the blood supply? Explain your answer.

11. The concentration of the dialysate used in peritoneal dialysis can vary (4.25%, 2.5%, 1.5% dextrose). How might the concentration of the dialysate affect the outcome?

12. Discuss fluid (water) movement in the following dialysis situations:

a.   dialysate more concentrated than blood

b.   dialysate less concentrated than blood

13. A client needs to undergo dialysis. Comment on the composition of the dialysate that could be used in the following situations:

a. client with concentration of water in the vascular compartment too high

b. water content in the blood too low (dehydration)

c. water content of blood at a normal level

d. client with a high sodium deficiency and fluctuations in daily intake.

Appendix 4: 'Science' laboratory sheet

Please Note:

This lab is designed in two sections. For the first component your *Lab coat* could be a valuable adjunct – or you could use the plastic aprons supplied if you have managed to sell the lab coat.

For the second component you should organise that the A&E notes for *Tom O'Hara* and *Magdalen O'Brien* are available within your group. Pharmacology, pathophysiology, physiology texts might also be useful.

Step 1

The session will start in the *wet lab* where there will be available for each group a *sheep's pluck* to examine, dissect and generally use to assist you to become more familiar with the respiratory and cardiac systems.

Come to this session with some plan of how to go about the dissection and some idea of the various components you would expect to be able to identify. Some notes to assist your exploration will be provided in the lab.

You may spend as much time as you require on the dissection.

Step 2

In the *nursing lab* there will be available the models of the *human heart* and *human torso* as well as various posters to try to assist you to contextualise what you have seen in the dissection with what is present in the living human body.

The computer program presenting simulated ECG measurements will also be available if you wish to revisit the electrical conduction system of the heart.

Step 3

In your groups consider again the information you have about the two clients *Tom O'Hara* (Unstable angina?) and *Magdalen O'Brien* (COAD and asthma).

(a) Relate the presenting symptoms to the anatomy/physiology of the major systems involved; both clients present with shortness of breath and sweatiness as component symptoms – what might this indicate?

(b) Consider the prescribed medications in terms of their effects on the physiology of the systems involved. NOTE – both clients are given oxygen as an adjunct to effect relief – what is the rationale here?

(c) Is oxygen a drug?
What are the major uses of oxygen therapy?
What are the various causes of hypoxia?
Are there some instances where oxygen therapy would be contraindicated? Explain.

Step 4

In your group consider in more detail the information you have for *Magdalen O'Brien*.

(a) Pulse – rapid, regular 108
Respiration – 32
BP – 120/79
What do these observations indicate?

(b) ABG 1 (on arrival) ABG 2 (some time later)

ABG 1 (on arrival)	ABG 2 (some time later)
pH 7.30	pH
PO_2 186	PO_2 156
PCO_2 60	PCO_2 49
HCO_3 30	HCO_3 28
BE 2.0	BE 2.4

What information can you deduce from the ABG analysis results above?

(c) Oxygen saturation SaO_2 99% – what does this indicate?

(d) What is the oxygen concentration of inspired air? Consider the oxygen therapy given to the client:

50% O_2 in ambulance
24% O_2 in accident and emergency
How is this treatment reflected in the ABG results?
Why is the client continued on O_2 when PO_2 is elevated and SaO_2 is 99%?

(e) Why might a sputum culture have been ordered?

(f) The following drugs have been mentioned in the notes.

  (i)   What are their actions in terms of effects on the respiratory system?
  (ii) Do they have effects on any other body system?
  (iii) To what class of drug does each belong?
      – Ventolin
      – Atrovent
      – Becloforte
      – Amoxil
      – Hydrocortisone.

Step 5

In your group consider in more detail the information you have for *Tom O'Hara*.

(a) Pulse 71–60
  Respiration 20
  BP 159/106–140/90

  Why might the client's BP have been so high when he first arrived in accident and emergency?

  The diastolic pressure remains relatively high an hour later – what might this indicate?

(b) Given that the client has diagnosed angina why consider JVP and chest X-ray results?

  Why have cardiac enzyme studies been requested?

(c) The following drugs have been mentioned in the notes or accompanying doctor's letter.

  (i)   What are their actions in terms of effects on the cardiac system?
  (ii) Do they have effects on any other body system?
  (iii) To what class of drug does each belong?
      – Aspirin
      – Anginine
      – Metoprolol
      – Transiderm
      – Diltiazem.

(d) (i) Given the client has diagnosed angina, why is he prescribed metoprolol?
   (ii) Why are headaches a common adverse effect of angina medication?

Step 6

For both clients an underlying concept is oxygen supply and compromise of oxygen supply to the tissues of the body. Explore this idea drawing parallels between the two situations and highlighting the differences. The following list may be useful.

oxygen transport	cardiac circulation
cardiac output	pulmonary circulation
gaseous exchange	systemic circulation
haemoglobin	tissue metabolism
ATP production	anoxia
hypoxia	ischaemia
infarction	

Appendix 5: Worksheet for learning package 1 (Module 2)

Audrey Faulkner and Terence Doherty

Questions 1–24 of this worksheet address the general concept of respiration. With a basic understanding in this area, you should be able to work your way through these questions identifying any specific learning needs which still require further attention to improve your knowledge base.

The questions from 25 on are more specific for this particular situation-improvement package and may serve as a guide to direct your inquiry processes.

1. List in order the structures that a molecule of oxygen from the atmosphere would pass in order to reach the bloodstream.
2. Continue the description of the course of events for this element to reach, for example, a skeletal muscle.
3. Explain what is meant by *external respiration*, *internal respiration* and *cellular respiration*.
4. How is air caused to enter the lungs?
5. How is air caused to leave the lungs?
6. What are the roles of *compliance*, *elastic recoil* and *surfactant* in ventilation?
7. Explain the physiological significance of *nasal hair*, *mucus* and *ciliary action* within the respiratory tract?
9. Why are the cartilages that reinforce the trachea C-shaped instead of full circles?
10. Describe the action of the major muscles involved in respiration during both inspiration and expiration.

11. During normal quiet breathing expiration is a passive process. This is not the case when breathing is greatly increased or when significant airway obstruction exists. Which muscles are the principal, accessory, expiratory muscles and what is their action?

12. The types of cells lining the respiratory tract vary dependent on the section of the tract. What are these various cell types, where in the tract are they found and what are their functions?

13. Discuss the pressure changes that occur during one respiratory cycle in terms of *intrapulmonary, intrapleural, alveolar* and *atmospheric*.

14. Define the following terms – *tidal volume, inspiratory volume, expiratory volume, residual volume, vital capacity, inspiratory capacity, functional residual capacity* and *total lung capacity*. Represent them diagrammatically.

15. Why is the size of the capillaries surrounding the alveoli important physiologically?

16. Explain oxygen and carbon dioxide movement in the circulatory system.

17. What is meant by *partial pressure* in respect to oxygen and carbon dioxide?

18. How can blood gas measurements be used to assess respiratory function?

19. What are the effects on oxygen–haemoglobin binding of changes in the following – *temperature, pH, partial pressure of carbon dioxide* and *concentration of DPG*.

20. Would you expect the concentration of HCO_3 to be greater in the plasma from an artery or a vein? Why?

21. During exercise, haemoglobin releases more oxygen to active skeletal muscle than when muscles are at rest. Why and how does this occur?

22. How would an obstruction of the airways affect the body's pH?

23. Breathing normally occurs at a regular rhythmic rate, but both rate and depth can be altered by neural and chemical signals. Discuss.

24. Smooth muscles of the bronchioles are under autonomic nervous system control. What are the differences between sympathetic and parasympathetic stimulation?

25. Five-year-old Billy suffers from recurrent bacterial pneumonias and chronic abdominal pain. He is underweight for his age and his skin has a dry, papery texture. Analysis of his perspiration reveals unusually high levels of sodium, potassium and chloride ion concentrations. What condition might Billy have? How are the symptoms related?

26. Cystic fibrosis is a genetic disorder classified as *autosomal recessive*. What does this mean? What are the other classes of genetic disorders?

27. Cystic fibrosis is a disorder of which body components?

28. What characterises the disorder and therefore what are the resultant signs, symptoms and implications?

29. Which is the most common organism causing recurrent infection in CF clients? (Give some background information)
30. What is your understanding of an opportunistic pathogen and how does this relate to infections in CF clients?
31. Comment on the *pharmacokinetics* and *pharmacodynamics* of the various drugs prescribed for Terence and Audrey. Include the various routes of administration, the combinations of drugs, synergistic action of drugs, types of drugs, etc.

Appendix 6: Facilitator guide (Dialysis experiment – lab Monday 3 August)

Terms

- *osmosis* – diffusion of a solvent across a membrane (in most cases in the physiological situation the solvent is water)
- *diffusion* – movement of molecules or ions from one region to another because of random molecular motion
- *osmolality* and *osmolarity* – virtually identical when water is the solvent – to express concentration of solute in terms of number of particles. For example, glucose does not dissociate in solution, hence 1 mole of glucose = 1 osmole, whereas sodium chloride does dissociate to give sodium ions and chloride ions, hence 1 mole of sodium chloride = 2 osmoles.

    (*molal* solution – 1 mole of *solute* in 1 kilogram of *solvent*
    molar solution – 1 mole of *solute* in 1 litre of *solvent*)

- *semi-permeable membrane* – membrane which allows the free passage of only certain molecules – may relate to size, shape, charge, etc.
- with reference to blood e.g.
- *hypertonic* – more concentrated (more solutes) hence movement of water from blood to the solution
- *hypotonic* – less concentrated, movement of water from solution to blood
- *isotonic/normotonic* – concentration the same as blood, dynamic equilibrium of water movement
- *filtration* – one-way process through a membrane involving *hydrostatic pressure* which forces liquid with ions and small molecules through membranes (leaves behind large molecules)
- *dialysis* – process of liquids, small molecules and ions passing through a membrane
- *dialysate* – dialysising solution – solution which forms the liquid on the side of the membrane opposite to the blood

Haemodialysis – blood passed on one side of an artificial semi-permeable membrane with a suitable dialysate on the other passing in the opposite direction. Involves *diffusion, osmosis* and *filtration*.

Peritoneal dialysis – the membranes are not artificial but are those surrounding the abdominal cavity. Involves *diffusion* and *osmosis*.

Experiment

Expected observations

1. iodine should move from beaker into the tubing – colour change in tubing to blue – beaker should remain yellow/brown
   water should move into tubing increasing size and firmness
   passive diffusion and osmosis to try to reach equilibrium
2. iodine should move from tubing to beaker – colour change in beaker to blue – tubing remains yellow
   possibly some water should move from tubing hence decrease in firmness
3. no colour movement or change but water should move into the tubing increasing firmness
4. blue colour (copper sulphate) should move out of tubing into beaker, water should move into the tubing giving a slight increase in firmness.

Trigger questions
(some clues to answers)

Starch molecules have a large molecular weight so cannot move across membrane. Iodine, water and copper sulphate are all of small molecular weight so exhibit free movement across membrane.

Starch-iodine complex has a large molecular weight therefore no movement should be seen. Students should realise that the movement of small substances can occur freely in both directions across the membrane.

In haemodialysis and peritoneal dialysis the membranes are porous enough to allow all constituents of plasma except plasma proteins to diffuse freely in both directions. Students should be able to identify the major components of plasma and discuss the changes that would occur to their concentrations on dialysis.

Basic objective is to remove from the blood excess or unwanted substances. These can be waste products, eg urea, creatinine, or excessive amounts of normal essential substances, eg electrolytes, acids, bases, glucose, water, or drugs, eg overdose barbiturates.

Second objective may be to increase the concentration in the blood of certain substances, eg electrolytes, water.

Cannot ever *totally* remove any substance in a dialysis process as the underlying principle is to equalise the concentrations across the membrane.

When considering the difference in concentration of dialysate used in peritoneal dialysis – 4.25% removes the largest amount of water from blood because of higher glucose concentration – this may also result in movement of glucose into the blood.

Quest 6
(a) water movement from blood to dialysate, ie removal of water from vascular compartment
(b) water movement into blood.

Quest 7
(a) dialysate more concentrated – hypertonic
(b) dialysate hypotonic – allow for water to move into the blood
(c) dialysate isotonic – no effective water movement
(d) add sodium to dialysate to facilitate uptake into vascular compartment.

Appendix 7: A study of students' perceptions of the anticipated and actual clinical experience in the first year of a Bachelor of Nursing

The study, undertaken in 1992, used students' experience of the clinical programme as the basis of a detailed description of all aspects of the clinical experience integrated within the degree. As well as a detailed description from students documenting anticipated and encountered difficult or challenging clinical situations, data were also sought regarding clinical facilitation and certain aspects of the problem-based course.

Data were gained from students before and after their series of hospital and community placements in Semester 2, Year 1. The data and discussion outlined relate to students' expectations and experiences about the effectiveness of eleven facilitation characteristics during clinical and the usefulness of certain aspects of the problem-based course in dealing with difficult or challenging clinical situations.

The clinical experience in Semester 1 of Year 1 focuses on health and wellness and incorporates health-related activities, such as health promotion sessions with adolescents, interviews with migrants and families, and investigations of health-related community resources. Semester 2 has a different focus, taking the themes of adaptation and loss and the consequences of these for individuals or groups. Students are thus placed in a series of four separate weeks of hospital or community settings for related clinical experiences.

Self-administered questionnaires were distributed to all available Year 1 students. (Pre-clinical questionnaires were distributed to all students who attended a pre-clinical information session and post-clinical questionnaires were distributed to all students who attended the last day of clinical practice for the year.) One hundred and five pre-clinical and one hundred and three post-clinical questionnaires were returned for analysis.

The analysis of the data in relation to facilitation characteristics and aspects of the course is essentially exploratory in nature and compares the mean scores of different age groups, and those with and without previous nursing experience. Comparisons are made between the before and after clinical findings and the different groups of students. The average scores were determined from the rank each student gave to each of the characteristics and aspects of the course.

In examining what students anticipated and experienced as effective clinical facilitation support in dealing with difficult or challenging situations, eleven facilitation characteristics were selected by the teaching staff from the guidelines in the Bachelor of Nursing submission document, as those elements that may be useful in facilitating learning in the clinical environment.

The eleven facilitation characteristics are:

1. Encourages student initiative
2. Provides guidance
3. Acknowledges student priorities
4. Actively talks with and listens to students
5. Clarifies learning contracts
6. Is available for consultation
7. Provides reassurance and support
8. Acknowledges the value of students' contribution
9. Provides time for reflection
10. Provides feedback through evaluation
11. Facilitates group functioning and maintenance.

Table 1 shows the pre-clinical and post-clinical mean scores for the comparison of facilitation characteristics. Average scores were determined from the rating each student gave to each of the eleven facilitator characteristics (with 0 = not effective and 5 = very effective) when asked, 'please indicate how effective you would find each of the following facilitation characteristics in assisting you to deal with difficult or challenging situations during clinical experiences' (pre-clinical); and 'Please indicate how effective you found each of the following facilitator characteristics in assisting you to deal with difficult or challenging situations during clinical experiences' (post-clinical).

Table 1: Comparison – average rating of facilitation characteristics – pre-clinical and post-clinical
(0 = not useful; 5 = very useful)

Facilitator	Total		Exp		No exp		Age gp: 17–20		Age gp: 21–30		Age gp: 31–50	
	Pre n = 105	Post n = 103	Pre (35)	Post (35)	Pre (70)	Post (66)	Pre (54)	Post (51)	Pre (33)	Post (37)	Pre (18)	Post (14)
Encourages student initiative	3.8	4.2	4.5	4.0	3.6	4.2	3.6	4.3	4.3	4.1	4.1	3.8
Provides guidance	4.3	4.1	4.6	3.9	4.3	4.3	4.2	4.3	4.5	4.1	4.5	3.7
Acknowledges student priorities	4.1	3.9	4.5	3.8	4.1	3.9	4.0	3.9	4.3	3.9	4.5	3.3
Actively talks with and listens to students	4.6	4.4	4.6	4.1	4.7	4.6	4.5	4.7	4.7	4.2	4.5	3.8
Clarifies learning contracts	4.0	3.8	4.5	3.4	3.9	4.0	3.8	4.2	4.1	3.6	4.4	3.0
Is available for consultation	4.3	4.0	4.4	3.7	4.3	4.1	4.5	4.2	4.3	3.7	4.3	3.8
Provides reassurance and support	4.6	4.2	4.6	4.0	4.6	4.4	4.5	4.5	4.4	4.0	4.8	4.0
Acknowledges the value of students' contribution	4.3	3.9	4.6	4.0	4.2	4.0	4.3	4.0	4.2	3.9	4.3	3.8
Provides time for reflection	4.1	3.9	4.4	3.6	4.0	4.2	3.8	4.2	4.2	3.7	4.5	3.5
Provides feedback through evaluation	4.1	4.1	4.4	3.8	4.1	4.2	4.0	4.3	4.1	4.1	4.6	3.2
Facilitates group functioning and maintenance	3.8	3.7	3.9	3.6	3.9	3.8	3.9	3.8	3.9	3.9	3.7	3.3

Eight aspects of the course were also listed for students to rank. These aspects represent the major elements of the problem-based course. A number of these elements reflect the problem-based tutorial process where students, 'guided by the facilitative skill of the tutor, engage in the process of making clinical judgments using systematic reasoning and integrating information from diverse fields' (Griffith University 1990:44).

The other elements reflect the strategies used to facilitate skill development within the problem-based learning strategy. The findings regarding certain aspects of the course emerge from data about the following:

1. Learning packages developed from real clinical situations
2. Working through nursing laboratory sheets for skill development
3. Nursing laboratory sheets are integrated within the context of the learning package and module focus
4. Being responsible for your own learning
5. Being able to apply the problem-solving skills used in processing the learning packages
6. Being able to apply the clinical reasoning skills used in processing the learning packages
7. Working co-operatively in a group
8. The Global Nursing Practice Assessment (GNPA)
9. Being able to have certain skills credentialled (assessed) on-campus

Table 2 shows the pre-clinical and post-clinical mean scores for each aspect of the course in relation to the questions; 'What aspects of the course do you believe will help you to deal with difficult or challenging clinical situations?' (pre-clinical); and 'What aspects of the course do you believe helped you to deal with difficult or challenging clinical situations?' (post-clinical). Ratings for aspects of the course were on the whole lower than those for facilitation characteristics, ranging from the lowest total average rank of 2.9 (not useful) for 'The Global Nursing Practice Assessment (GNPA)' (post-clinical) to the highest 4.0 (very useful) for 'Being able to apply the clinical reasoning skills used in the processing of the LPs', 'Working co-operatively in a group' (pre-clinical) and 'Being able to have certain skills credentialled (assessed) on-campus' (post-clinical).

Appendix 8: Student responses to learning packages

The process for surveying student perceptions of the learning packages they were undertaking was established by agreement between facilitators and a member of the university's higher education centre assisting in the evaluation.

Table 2: Comparison – average rating of aspects of the course for total populations – pre-clinical and post-clinical
(0 = not useful; 5 = very useful)

Aspects of the course	Total		Exp		No exp		Age gp: 17–20		Age gp: 21–30		Age gp: 31–50	
	Pre n = 105	Post n = 103	Pre (35)	Post (35)	Pre (70)	Post (66)	Pre (54)	Post (51)	Pre (33)	Post (37)	Pre (18)	Post (14)
Learning packages developed from 'real' clinical situations	3.7	3.4	3.8	3.7	3.6	3.3	3.7	3.3	3.8	3.8	3.7	3.0
Working through nursing laboratory sheets for skill development	3.7	3.2	3.4	2.9	3.7	3.4	3.7	3.2	3.8	3.3	3.8	3.4
Nursing laboratory sheets are integrated within the context of the learning package and module focus	3.9	3.5	3.8	3.4	3.9	3.5	4.6	3.3	3.8	3.7	4.0	3.3
Being responsible for your own learning	3.5	3.7	3.6	4.1	3.5	3.5	3.4	3.6	3.9	4.1	3.5	3.5
Being able to apply the problem-solving skills used in processing learning packages	3.9	3.5	4.2	3.7	3.7	3.4	3.6	3.5	4.2	3.8	3.7	3.1
Being able to apply the clinical reasoning skills used in processing learning packages	4.0	3.7	4.1	3.8	4.0	3.6	3.9	3.5	4.1	3.9	4.2	3.6
Working co-operatively in a group	4.0	3.5	4.1	3.4	4.0	3.6	4.0	3.6	4.3	3.6	3.7	3.0
The Global Nursing Practice	3.2	2.9	3.0	2.6	3.2	3.1	3.1	2.9	3.3.	3.0	3.4	2.7
Being able to have certain skills credentialled (assessed) on-campus		4.0		3.9		4.1		3.9		4.0		4.5

The facilitator of each problem-based tutorial group explained the process to students in the group, and handed to a volunteer student a number of evaluation questionnaires and envelopes. The task of this student was to collect completed questionnaires from students without the facilitator seeing the completed forms, to seal the questionnaires in a given envelope and to mail it in the university's internal system to the member concerned in the higher education centre. The purpose of this procedure was to encourage full and frank expression of views from students.

The questionnaires were then processed, and the results forwarded only to the facilitator of the group who had completed the survey. It was then up to the facilitator to make use of the results in whatever way the facilitator thought appropriate. In most cases this included sharing the results with students, and discussing the results with colleagues during reflection sessions on learning packages.

The questionnaire itself comprised four items: 1) 'What in your view were the best features of the learning package?' 2) 'What in your view were the worst features of the learning package?' 3) 'What changes would you make to the learning package?' and 4) 'If you would like to make other comments please give them here'. Responses were categorised broadly with frequencies of response, as well as being listed verbatim under each questionnaire item. A covering note accompanied the results returned to each facilitator.

Below is an example of what a facilitator would receive; this is an actual case, reproduced in full (meanings of some of the responses will be obscure to readers, but of course they made sense to the facilitator concerned who was familiar with what the students would have been referring to).

Covering note accompanying result of 'Student Responses to Learning Packages'

Dear [tutor's name]   15 April 91

Enclosed is information concerning student response to learning package 2. I'd like to mention some points about it:

The information concerns only the students in your group for the learning package indicated. The information was taken from questionnaires entitled 'Student response to learning package' which, you'll recall, students completed near the end of the learning package indicated.

The information is provided in two forms:

(a) First, by broad category; i.e., where students made broadly similar comments these were placed in the same category. The number of responses in each category is given for your group. The purpose of this broad categorisation is to summarise the information in a way which may be helpful.

If you have any suggestions as to a set of categories you might find more helpful, or if you would find it helpful for the present categories to be modified, please let me know.

(b) The second list contains all the responses the students in your group made, typed out verbatim, except where students mentioned someone other than yourself by name. If someone else was mentioned the comment has been removed and passed on only to the person concerned. The exception to this is: if the mention of a name was only for reference (e.g., 'we covered the respiratory system in J. Smith's fixed resource session') then it has been left in. One comment was removed from your list.

In some cases it is easy to identify individuals even though they are not mentioned by name. I've tried to use appropriate discretion in these cases, but if you have any concerns about the result please do discuss it with me so that we can seek a better arrangement.

Interpretation and action. In the past (in other degree programmes) student responses of this sort have sometimes been treated as final conclusions. It is very important to note that in some respects this is a mistake. Two examples may help clarify this. One, suppose many students say 'I did not understand such and such a journal article for the learning package and still do not'. It would be reasonable to regard that as a conclusion that calls for change of some kind – e.g., by changing the article, or by finding ways of explaining it so that students could understand it.

Second, suppose many students say 'The facilitator was not directive', and intend this as a complaint. This is quite different from the first example. If the educational point of facilitation is to help students become self-directive, then arguably the facilitator's non-directiveness is a good thing and ought not to be changed. Whether or not the actual facilitation does or does not need changing to be more helpful is a question that the facilitator may need to consider. However, the student comment *alone* is not sufficient ground to make any change.

In the past, too, student responses have sometimes been dismissed because they conflict – some students say something was the best feature, and others say it was the worst. However, dismissal of conflicting comments may be too hasty, since the reasons students have for responding in this way can be revealing. Unfortunately, brief questionnaires usually don't yield the reasons, but other information in the responses together with one's own reflection on the learning package and responses to it can result in a useful appraisal of the responses.

Overall, the general point is that the comments *need interpretation and reflection* in order to decide whether any change is needed.

If you have questions about this, or would like to discuss anything with me, please get in touch.

Best wishes

Don

Results of 'Student Responses to Learning Packages'

[The following responses were made by Year 1 students in a problem-based tutorial group (comprising around eighteen students) within the first few weeks of their studies; the learning package they were commenting on was the second that they had undertaken.]

(a) Broad categories of student responses

What in your view were the BEST features of the learning package?

Rank		No. of student responses
1	Knowledge	12
2	Learning methods	10
3	Relevance	4
4	Resources	3
5	Content	2
6	Questionnaire	1
	Communication skills	1

What in your view were the WORST features of the learning package?

1	Repetition	13
2	Course duration	3
3	Information	2
	Satisfactory [no worst features]	2
4	Questionnaire	1
	Learning	1

What CHANGES would you make to the learning package?

1	Timing/duration	6
2	No changes	5
3	Repetition	4

4	Question changes	3
5	Information	2
6	Content	1
	Block 2	1

If you would like to make any other comments please give them here
| 1 | Other | 4 |

(b) Verbatim student responses

1. What in your view were the BEST features of the learning package?

We as a group were able to pool our knowledge skills and resources to produce a poster and teaching format aimed at 15-year-old high school students about our topic transmission of STDs [sexually transmitted diseases].

It makes students make an effort to do the research work and be co-operative in class and not just as a single student. Makes them more analytical and resourceful.

The getting together as a group – assimilation of ideas.

The Belbin Questionnaire was an excellent way of sorting out any confusion. It brought about a better understanding of myself as well as others in the Group. I consider we work well together.

It really made us look into the period of 'adolescence' and appreciate the problems that have to be dealt with. It was a good way to learn about men and women. Reproductive organs and pregnancy, STDs and contraception. It all flowed together well.

The best features of the learning package were the discussion groups because every angle of the problem was brought to attention. Also the biological lectures and the sexuality lectures also were useful in a way.

The reality of the problem discussed in the learning package.

The wide range of resources available for that problem.

The relevance of the learning package in 'today's' society.

The problems were real problems that do happen. It was good to have a real problem to deal with. I did learn from this learning package and Learning Package 1.

I opened up a lot of issues that needed looking into. Health nurse discussing about adolescent sexuality.

Open discussion and learning tutorials.

Collecting information from all different resources, using our own initiative.

Self-directed learning really makes you think so the information we research really sinks in.

Sessions with [tutor's name]. Group discussions about Anthea's problems and the issues surrounding this. [Anthea was the name of the client in the learning package.]

The best features of the learning package were the ways that we had to go out and research a lot of the facts. This in fact helped me to understand better, and that I was learning and as a result, I am not left confused. I also liked the fact that it left a lot of options and so we could look at a lot of different aspects of Anthea's problem.

It is a real life situation that could actually happen to us when we are working.

It encouraged lateral thinking which is very good.

Researching for a better understanding of how, if we were school health nurses, we would help someone in Anthea's situation.

Enjoyed the biological input also very much enjoyed the law lecture. Family Planning was excellent as well as microbiology and communication or some parts of it.

Very informative.

All information given was useful to the learning package.

Communication skills were good.

Resources were good – policeman, school health nurse, etc.

It made you stop and think about what you could do if you or a friend were in that situation. Finding out about the various services involved was very interesting.

We learnt a lot about the role of the School Health Nurse and there was plenty of information there if we were interested and keen. I found there were a few things that I didn't know about until then.

The discussion on the legalities of under age sex and just finding out how many people a 15-year-old girl (presumably pregnant) can go to. STDs was interesting.

The role of the School Nurse. Legal and Ethical issues.

Growth and development of adolescents.

2. *What in your view were the WORST features of the learning package?*

None! More information regarding adolescent development and anatomy is up to our own personal study; the basic information was given, it was up to us to expand on the information.

If the student is lazy and dependent, he/she will not learn.

Repetition Hearing many things over and over.

An example is contraception and diseases for instance AIDS in book – pamphlets – role-play – lecture.

The second block really seemed to have been covered in the first week and I felt that we were going over and over the same things.

Repetition of some viewpoints of the actual learning package and issues involved in it.

The repeating of questions and ideas in Block 2.

The questions especially in Block 2 seem to cover one question, e.g. you'll answer one question and then go on to the next and we found the question covered the above answers.

Some of the information was gone over a few times.

Family planning discussion tutorial in the cinema was a waste of time. Most of us had already gathered the information in the week before that tutorial.

More biology (anatomy and physiology) tutorials are still needed. We are still not getting enough 'formal' information.

Block 2 was repeating itself quite a lot or it repeated what we had already done previously in the learning package.

The worst features of the learning package would be the fact that we kept on going over a lot of things. What I mean is that a lot of the questions were very repetitive. Some of the questions were a repeat of other questions, just worded differently.

The learning package seemed to drag on. I feel there wasn't really enough there for the full 2 weeks, especially in the second half of the learning package.

There wasn't enough information e.g. we didn't know anything about her boyfriend so we had to interpret ourselves what her boyfriend might have been like.

Felt the repetition at the end of the learning package. e.g. Seemed to be summarising too much. Contraception and sex education was also repetitious.

Did not like the questionnaire Belbin Team Role as I feel it isn't very accurate as people present differently to different situations.

Towards the end it seemed to drag on.

It was dragged out too long. The whole learning package could have been finished in one week. By the second week, everyone was getting sick of it, and no-one was interested. The questions in Block 2 were a waste of time, because they all seemed to be asking the same thing.

Some of the questions were repeating previous questions or receiving previous questions which felt like a bit of a waste of time.

Having to listen to the Family Planning talk on Thursday when in fact it had already been covered in our talk with [tutor's name]. The repetition of particular issues became monotonous.

There was not that I could recall.

3. *What CHANGES would you make to the learning package?*

I feel the learning package went well, I enjoyed striving towards my personal aims with my peers.

I like the learning package, I don't think it would need to be changed.

I am happy with the way the learning packages are being implemented.

I would have preferred to have the family planning lecture earlier on in the learning package.

Perhaps the second block in the learning package could have had maybe a different question so as the repetition of ideas may not have occurred, otherwise nothing.

The only change I would make is in Block 2. I would either cut it completely out or use other means to portray the info. given in it.

More direct questions.

No response.

More concrete information given.

Help from the facilitator to put us on a definite tack at the beginning of the learning package.

Having Family Planning Session before assessment piece was finished.

I would like to change the learning package by maybe not dragging so long on the learning packages. This learning package in particular kept dragging on with the same questions all the time.

Reduce the amount of time available for the students to work on the learning package. I don't think the full 2 weeks was required to finish the learning package.

I would write something about Anthea's boyfriend.

Would like to see more Biology I think. Not much repetition.

Maybe shorten it a bit.

Make it into a one week learning package, so everyone remains interested in what they are doing.

Just some of the questions that's all.

Just not too much repetition of particular issues i.e. adolescents were done to death.

None.

4. *If you would like to make any other comments please give them here:*

Overall a really great way of learning.

No more 'Exam pressure'.

I would like to see not so much work done with butcher paper. Although I cannot think of a better suggestion at this time.

There seemed to be some repetition on most issues, probably more than necessary.

Appendix 9: Student attitudes to facilitating – Semester 1, 1993

Some facilitators used the 'Student responses to learning packages' questionnaire, but with students asked to comment on facilitation rather than on the learning packages. A questionnaire specifically for obtaining information on facilitation, 'Student Attitudes to Facilitating – Semester 1, 1993', was developed by staff in the nursing programme in consultation with staff in the higher education centre.

It comprised four sections. The first contained eighteen statements with responses on a five-point scale, and a nineteenth with a response on a seven-point scale. The second and third sections contained one item each, with responses on a seven-point scale. The statements, and the response scales, are given below. Results in the form of means and standard deviations for each item were reported to the facilitator concerned, together with the percentage of responses to each of the response-points 1–5 and 0. The fourth section allowed for open-ended responses. Questionnaires were returned to the facilitator at the end of the semester so that open-ended responses could be read.

Section 1

Response scale for first eighteen items:

1 Strongly Agree	2 Agree	3 Uncertain	4 Disagree	5 Strongly Disagree	0 N/A

Items:

Please read each of the statements below and circle the number on the response scale which corresponds most closely to your experience of this staff member's facilitation in your tutorial group.

1. The staff member maintains a student centred focus
2. The staff member facilitates a supportive learning environment
3. The staff member helps the groups to learn co-operatively
4. The staff member is able to assist the group to resolve problems which may have disrupted group processes
5. The staff member facilitates tutorials in a way which encourages active learning
6. The staff member challenges students to provide evidence of critical reflection in relation to decision making

7. The staff member encourages students to analyse and synthesise new learning material
8. The staff member promotes the integration of clinical and theoretical learning
9. The staff member facilitates problem-based tutorial to maximise student learning
10. The staff member avoids providing 'right' answers
11. The staff member draws on students' previous experiences for examples and illustrations
12. The staff member encourages all students to express their own opinion
13. The staff member values students' contributions to group processes
14. The staff member helped me to learn independently
15. The staff member seemed willing to offer individual help
16. The staff member made the assessment requirements clear
17. Assessment items are returned promptly
18. The staff member provides helpful feedback on group and individual assignments

Response scale for items 19 and 20

I Very Poor	2	3	4	5	6	7 Outstanding	0 No Answer

Section 3

Items:

19. In general, how would you rate *Nursing Programme* this semester?

    This question asks about the staff member's *overall effectiveness in facilitating learning in your tutorial group*. Please disregard your feelings about the Programme and focus your attention on the way in which this staff member uses facilitation.
20. All things considered, how would you rate this staff member's overall effectiveness in facilitation?

Section 4

Items:

(PLEASE PRINT YOUR ANSWERS TO PRESERVE ANONYMITY)

The questionnaire will be returned to staff members for their perusal after assessment for this semester has been completed.

21. What were the staff member's strengths in facilitation?
22. What improvements would you suggest?

Thank you for your help

Appendix 10: Main results of a Year 3 survey

Towards the end of their studies in the third year, students were surveyed twice by questionnaire. Main results of the Course Experience Questionnaire were given in the main text.

Below, main results are given of a questionnaire drawn up by staff in the programme. It had two parts, the first seeking written responses to various items. The second part, for which results are given below, sought responses on a five-point scale, as indicated. The number of students responding to the survey was 108 (a response rate of approximately 80%). Questionnaire items and results:

Please indicate how effective you found each of the following facilitator characteristics in Year 3 in assisting you to develop enquiry and critical thinking skills; clinical reasoning, problem-solving and self-evaluation.

Not effective					Very effective	N/A
0	1	2	3	4	5	

	Mean
Encouraged student initiative	4.0
Provided guidance	3.7
Acknowledged student priorities	3.2
Actively talked with and listened to students	3.3
Promoted mutual respect	3.9
Provided a supportive learning environment	3.9
Assisted students to self-evaluate	3.7
Acknowledged the value of students' contribution	3.8
Provided time for reflection	3.9
Provided feedback through evaluation	4.0
Facilitated group functioning and maintenance	4.0

What aspects of the Year 3 course have you found useful in facilitating your learning?

Not effective					Very effective	N/A
0	1	2	3	4	5	

	Mean
Situation Improvement Packages (learning packages) developed from real clinical situations	3.4
Working through nursing laboratory sheets for skill development	4.3
Nursing laboratory sheets are integrated within the context of the learning package and module focus	3.4
Being responsible for your own learning	3.8
Being able to apply the problem-solving skills used in processing learning packages	3.7
Being able to apply the clinical reasoning skills used in processing learning packages	4.1
Working co-operatively in a group	4.0
Small-group science tutorials	4.1
Being able to have certain skills credentialled (assessed) on-campus	4.2

Bibliography

Abrahamson, S. (1987) 'Harvard Medical School Tries a Problem-based Curriculum', *Chronical of Higher Education*, 34(8): B1–2.

Adkison, L. R. and Volpe, E. P. (1992) 'Advantages of a PBL Approach in Teaching Genetics', *Academic Medicine*, 67(11): 764.

Andersson, F. and Wallin, V. (1991) 'Student Impressions of Problem-based Learning', *EDS-Magazine*, 3(3): 14–15.

Barrows, H. S. (1976) 'An Evaluation of Problem-based Learning in Small Groups Utilising a Simulated Patient', *Journal of Medical Education*, 51(1): 52–4.

—— (1986) 'A Taxonomy of Problem-based Learning Methods', *Medical Education*, 20(6): 481–6.

—— (1988) *The Tutorial Process*, Springfield, Illinois: Southern Illinois University, School of Medicine.

Barrows, H. S. and Tamblyn, R. M. (1980) *Problem-based Learning: An Approach to Medical Education*, New York: Springer.

Biggs, J. B. (1989) 'Approaches to the Enhancement of Tertiary Teaching', *Higher Education Research and Development*, 8(1): 7–25.

Biran, L. A. (1991) 'Self-assessment and Learning through GOSCE (Group Objective Structured Clinical Examination)', *Medical Education*, 25(6): 475–9.

Birch, W. (1986) 'Towards a Model for Problem-based Learning', *Studies in Higher Education*, 11(1): 73–82.

Blainey, C. 1980 'Anxiety in the Undergraduate Medical – Surgical Clinical Student', *Journal of Nursing Education*, 19, 8: 33–6.

Boud, D. (1985) *Problem-based Learning in Education for the Professions*, Sydney: Higher Education Research and Development Society of Australasia.

—— (1986) 'Facilitating Learning in Continuing Education: Some Important Sources', *Studies in Higher Education*, 113: 237–43.

Boud, D. and Feletti, G. (eds) (1991) *The Challenge of Problem-based Learning*, London: Kogan Page.

Boud, D. and Griffin, V. (eds) (1987) *Appreciating Adult Learning – From the Learners' Perspective*, London: Kogan Page.

Boud, D. J., Keogh, R. and Walker, D. (eds) (1985) *Reflection: Turning Experience Into Learning*, London: Kogan Page.

Brockett, R. G. and Hiemstra, R. (1991) *Self Direction in Adult Learning: Perspectives on Theory, Research and Practice*, London: Routledge.

Brookfield, S. (1986) *Understanding and Facilitating Adult Learning*, San Francisco, California: Jossey-Bass.

Candy, P. C. (1991) *Self-direction in Lifelong Learning*, San Francisco, California: Jossey-Bass.

Cawley, P. (1989) 'The Introduction of a Problem-based Option into a Conventional Engineering Degree Course', *Studies in Higher Education*, 14: 83–95.

Chen, S. E. (1991) 'Profile of an Integrated Problem-based Architecture Course. Students' Perceptions and Preferences. The Technology of Design', *Proceedings of 1991 ANZA School of Architecture Conference*, Adelaide: 175–87.

Clarke, R. M. (1978) 'Problem-oriented Medical Education', *Proceedings of the Seventh Australian Medical Records Conference*, (18–21 May 1978) Australian National University.

—— (1981) 'A New Style of Undergraduate Curriculum: The Newcastle Experience and What it has to Offer', *ANZAME Bulletin*, October: 16–22.

Colby, K. *et al.* (1986) 'Problem-based Learning of Social Sciences and Humanities by Fourth-year Medical Students', *Journal of Medical Education*, 61(5): 413–15.

Colditz, G. A. (1980) 'The Students' View of an Innovative Undergraduate Medical Course: The First Year at the University of Newcastle, NSW', *Medical Education*, 14: 320–5.

Cordeiro, P. (1990) 'Problem-based Thematic Instruction', *Language-Arts*, 67(1): 26–34.

Creedy, D. and Horsfall, J. (1992) 'Problem-based Learning in Nurse Education: An Australian View', *Journal of Advanced Nursing*, 17(6): 727–33.

Dan Langenberghe, H. V. K. (1988) 'Evaluation of Students' Approaches to Studying in a Problem-based Physical Therapy Curriculum', *Journal of the American Physical Therapy Association*, 68(4): 522.

Des Marchais, J. E. (1991) 'From Traditional to Problem-based Curriculum: How the Switch was Made at Sherbrooke, Canada', *The Lancet*, 338.

—— (1993) 'A Student-centred, Problem-based Curriculum: 5 Years' Experience', *Canadian Medical Association Journal*, 148(9): 1567–72.

Des Marchais, J. E., Bureau, M. A., Dumais, B. and Pigeon, G. (1992) 'From Traditional to Problem-based Learning: A Case Report of Complete Curriculum Reform', *Medical Education*, 26: 190–9.

Eisenstaedt, R. S. *et al.* (1990) 'Problem-based Learning: Cognitive Retention and Cohort Traits of Randomly Selected Participants and Decliners', *Academic Medicine*, 65(9), suppl: S11–12.

Engel, C. (1991) 'Not Just a Method but a Way of Learning', in D. Boud and G. Feletti (eds) *The Challenge of Problem-Based Learning*, London: Kogan Page.

—— (1992) 'Problem-based Learning', *British Journal of Hospital Medicine*, 48(6): 325–9.

Engel, C. E., Clarke, R. M. and Feletti, G. I. (1982) 'The Evolution and Impact of Programme Evaluation in a New Medical School', *Assessment and Evaluation in Higher Education*, 7(3): 257–68.

Engel, C., Schmidt, H. and Vluygen, P. (eds) (1990) 'Students' Perceptions After One Year of Problem-based Learning at Sherbrooke', *Annals of the Network of Community Oriented Education, Vol. 3*. Maastricht: Network Secretariat, Rijksuniversiteit Limburg.

Entwistle, H. (1970) *Child-Centred Education*, London: Methuen.

Feletti, G. (1988) 'Problem-based Teaching and Learning', *ANZAME Bulletin*, 15(1): 57.

—— (1990) 'Trying Problem-based Learning in More Traditional Settings: What Seems to Work', *ANZAME Bulletin*, 17(3): 26–32.

Fisher, L. A. (1991) 'Evaluating the Impact of Problem-Based Learning: On the Institution and on Faculty', in D. Boud and G. Feletti (eds) *The Challenge of Problem-based Learning*, London: Kogan Page.

Friedman, R. de Blieck, Sheps, C. G., Greer, D. S., Mennin, S. P., Norman, G. R., Woodward, C. A. and Swanson, D. B. (1992) 'Charting the Winds of Change: Evaluating Innovative Medical Curricula', *Annals of Community-Oriented Medicine*, 5: 167–79.

Gibbs, G. (1992) *Improving the Quality of Student Learning*, Bristol: Technical and Education Services.

Glick, S. M. (1991) 'Problem-based Learning and Community Oriented Medical Education', *Medical Education*, 25(6): 542–5.

Gordon, M. and Winsor, K. (1988) *Report on Problem-based Learning and its Relevance to the Practical Legal Training Course*, St Leonards, New South Wales, Australia: College of Law.

Grady, C. (1984) 'In Defence of the Integrated Curriculum', *Journal of Nursing Education*, 23(7): 322–3.

Griffith University (1988a) *A Submission to the Queensland Minister for Health for the Establishment of a School of Nursing at Griffith University*, Division of Science and Technology.

Griffith University (1988b) Nursing Studies Planning Group, Minutes of Meeting 2/88.

Griffith University (1989) Nursing Studies Planning Group, Minutes of Meeting 3/89.

Griffith University (1990) *Bachelor of Nursing*, Brisbane: Griffith University.

Grol, R. *et al.* (1989) 'Effects of the Vocational Training of General Practice Consultation Skills and Medical Performance', *Medical Education*, 23(6): 512–21.

Hammond, M. and Collins, R. (1991) *Self-directed Learning: Critical Practice*, London: Kogan Page.

Heale, J., Davis, D., Norman, G., Woodward, C., Neufeld, V. and Dodd, P. (1988) 'A Randomised Controlled Trial Assessing the Impact of Problem-based Versus Didactic Teaching Methods in CME', *Proceedings of the 27th Annual Conference on Research in Medical Education*, Association of American Medical Colleges, Washington: 72–7.

Hengstberger-Sims, C. and McMillan, M. (1993) 'Problem-based Learning Packages: Considerations for Neophyte Package Writers', *Nurse Education Today*, 13: 73–7.

Hiemstra, R. (ed.) (1991) *Creating Environments for Effective Adult Learning: New Directions for Adult and Continuing Education*, San Francisco, California: Jossey-Bass.

Horsburgh, M., Lynes, L. and Oliver, L. O. (1984) 'Problem-based Learning: An Educational Strategy', *New Zealand Nursing Journal*, 77(8): 6–8.

Jones, D. (1978) 'The Need For a Comprehensive Counselling Service for Nursing Students', *Journal of Advanced Nursing*, 3: 359–68.

Kanitsaki, O. and Sellick, K. (1989) 'Clinical Nurse Teaching: An Investigation of Student Perceptions of Clinical Nurse Teacher Behaviours', *The Australian Journal of Advanced Nursing*, 6(4): 18–24.

Kaufmann, A. (1985) (ed.) *Implementing Problem-based Medical Education: Lessons from Successful Innovations*, New York: Springer.

Kaufmann, A. *et al.* (1989) 'The New Mexico Experiment: Educational Innovation and Institutional Change', *Academic Medicine*, 64(6): 285–94.

Kingston, G. and Mercer, T. (1987) *Problem-based Learning in Electronics*, Hawthorn, Victoria, Australia: Hawthorn Institute of Education.

Kjellgren, K., Ahlner, J., Dahlgren, L. O. and Haglund, L. (eds) (1993) *Problembaserad inlaring. Erfarenheter fran Halsouniverseitetet*, Lund: Studentlitteratur.

Kleehammer, K., Hart, L. and Fogel Keck, J. (1990) 'Nursing Students' Perceptions of Anxiety-Producing Situations in the Clinical Setting', *Journal of Nursing Education*, 29(4): 31–5.

Lewis, K. E. and Tamblyn, R. M. (1987) 'The Problem-based Learning Approach in Baccalaureate Role Nursing: How Effective is it?', *Nursing Papers*, 19(2): 17–26.

Little, P. J. (1986) *Problem-based Learning: a Staff Leave Report on Problem-based Learning in the Nursing and Medical Professions in the USA, Canada and New Zealand*, University of Western Sydney, Macarthur: unpublished report.

Little, P. J. and Ryan, G. L. (1988) 'Educational Change through Problem Learning', *Australian Journal of Advanced Nursing*, 5(4): 31–5.

Little, S. E. and Margetson, D. B. (1989) 'A Project-based Approach to Information Systems Design for Undergraduates', *The Australian Computer Journal*, 21(2): 130–8.

Little, S. E. and Sauer, C. (1991) 'Organizational and Institutional Impediments to a Problem-Based Approach', in D. Boud and G. Feletti (eds) *The Challenge of Problem-Based Learning*, London: Kogan Page.

McDermott, J. F. Jr and Anderson, A. S. (1991) 'Retraining Faculty for the Problem-based Curriculum at the University of Hawaii, 1989–1991', *Academic Medicine*, 66(12): 778–9.

McMillan, M. and Dwyer, J. (1988) 'Changing Times, Changing Paradigm (1): The Macarthur Experience', *Nursing Education Today*, 9(1): 93–9.

Margetson, D. B. (1987) 'The Question-led Design of a Degree Programme', *Higher Education Research and Development*, 6(2): 151–73.

—— (1989a) 'Is Problem-based Learning for the Professions Technicist?', *Research and Development in Higher Education*, 11: 145–9.

—— (1989b) 'Nursing Studies: Development of Planning', papers for 1/89 meeting of Nursing Studies Planning Group, Brisbane: Griffith University.

—— (1991) 'Is there a Future for Problem-based Education?', *Higher Education Review*, 23(2): 33–47.

—— (1993) 'Understanding Problem-based Learning', *Educational Philosophy and Theory*, 25(1): 40–57.

—— (1993) 'More Quality, Less Pedagogy: Understanding, Knowledge, and Problem-based Learning', presentation at the Higher Education Research and Development Society of Australasia, Brisbane.

—— (1994) 'Current Education Reform and the Significance of Problem-based Learning', *Studies in Higher Education* (in press).

Mattern, W. (1992) 'Should Faculty Tutors for PBL Groups be Content Experts?', *Academic Medicine*, 67(7): 454.

Mennin, S. P. and Martinez-Burrola, N. (1990) 'The Cost of Problem-based vs Traditional Medical Education', *Medical Education*, 20(3): 187–94.

Metsemakers, J. F., Bouhijs, P. A. and Snellen-Balendong, H. A. (1991) 'Do We Teach What We Preach? Comparing the Contents of Problem-based Medical Curriculum with Primary Health Care Data', *Family Practice*, 8(3): 195–201.

Midgley, M. (1991) *Wisdom, Information and Wonder: What is Knowledge for*, London: Routledge.

Mitchell, G. (1988) 'Problem-based Learning in Medical Schools: A New Approach', *Medical Teacher*, 10(1): 57–67.

Moust, J. C. and Nuy, H. J. (1987) 'Preparing Teachers for a Problem-based Student-centred Law Course', *The Journal of Professional Legal Education*, 5: 16–30.

Moust, J. H. C., De Volder, M. L. and Nuy, H. J. P. (1989) 'Peer Teaching and Higher Level Cognitive Outcomes in Problem-based Learning', *Higher Education*, 18: 737–42.

Neame, R. L. B. (1981) 'How to Construct a Problem-based Course', *Medical Teacher*, 3: 94–9.

—— (1982) 'Academic Roles and Satisfaction in a Problem-based Curriculum', *Studies in Higher Education*, 7(2): 141–51.

Nooman, Z. M., Schmidt, H. G. and Ezzat, E. S. (eds) (1990) *Innovation in Medical Education: An Evaluation of its Present Status*, New York: Springer.

Norman, G. R. (1988) 'Problem-solving Skills, Solving Problems and Problem-based Learning', *Medical Education*, 22(4): 279–86.

—— (1989) 'Problem-solving Skills Versus Problem-based Learning', *Cornell Vet*, 79: 4.

Norman, G. R. and Schmidt, H. G. (1992) 'The Psychological Basis of Problem-based Learning: A Review of the Evidence', *Academic Medicine*, 67(9): 557–65.

O'Shea, H. and Parsons, M. (1979) 'Clinical Instruction: Effective and Ineffective Teacher Behaviours', *Nursing Outlook*, June: 411–15.

Ostwald, M. J., Chen, S. E., Varnam, B. and McGeorge, D. (1992) *The Application of Problem-based Learning to Distance Education*, paper presented at the ICDE 16th International Conference, Bangkok, Thailand.

Ramsden, P. (1992) *Learning to Teach in Higher Education*, London: Routledge.

Rankin, J. A. (1992) 'Problem-based Medical Education: Effect on Library Use', *Bulletin of Medical Library Association*, 80(1): 36–43.

Rohlin, M. and Klinge, B. (1991) 'The "Malmo-model": A New Approach to the Undergraduate Dental Education at Lund University, Sweden', *EDS-Magazine*, 3(3): 7–13.

Rosen, R. L., Paul, H. A. and Goodman, L. J. (1992) 'Using a Database to Analyse Core Basic Science Content in a Problem-based Curriculum', *Academic Medicine*, 67(8): 535–8.

Rouse, M. W. (1990) 'Problem-based Learning: An Alternative to Traditional Education', *Journal of Optometric Education*, 15(4): 111–12.

Ryan, G. (1993) 'Student Perceptions About Self-directed Learning in a Professional Course Implementing Problem-based Learning', *Studies in Higher Education*, 18(1): 53–63.

Scheiman, M. and Whittaker, S. (1990) 'Implementing Problem-based Learning in the Didactic Curriculum', *Journal of Optometric Education*, 15(4): 113–18.

Schmidt, H. G. (1983) 'Problem-based Learning: Rationale and Description', *Medical Education*, 17: 11–16.

Schmidt, H. G. and Valdes, M. V. (eds) (1983) *Tutorials on Problem-based Learning*, Assen, The Netherlands: Van Gorcum.

Schmidt, H. G., Dauphnee, W. D. and Patel, V. L. (1987) 'Comparing the Effects of Problem-based and Conventional Curricula in an International Sample', *Medical Education*, 62(4): 305–15.

Scriven, M. (1981) *Evaluation Thesaurus* 3rd ed., Inverness, California: Edgepress.

Selleck, T. (1982) 'Satisfying and Anxiety-Creating Incidents for Nursing Students', *Nursing Times*, 1 December: 137–40.

Senge, P. M. (1990) 'The Leader's New Work: Building Learning Organisations', *Sloan Management Review*, Fall: 7–23.

Shahabndin, S. H. (1987) 'Content Coverage in Problem-based Learning', *Medical Education*, 21(4): 310–13.

Silver, M. and Wilkerson, L. (1992) 'Effects of Tutors with Subject Expertise on the Problem-based Tutorial Process', *Academic Medicine*, 66: 298–300.

Skipper, J. K. *et al.* (1989) 'Benefits of Hindsight: Design Problems in Evaluating Innovation in Medical Education', *Evaluation Practice*, 10(3): 7–11.

Thompson, D. G. and Williams, R. G. (1985) 'Barriers to the Acceptance of Problem-based Learning in Medical Schools', *Studies in Higher Education*, 10(2): 199–204.

van der Vleuten, C. and Wijnen, W. (eds) (1990) *Problem-based Learning: Perspectives from the Maastricht approach*, Amsterdam: Thesis Press.

Vernon, D. T., Campbell, J. D. and Dally, J. C. (1992) 'Problem-based Learning in Two Behavioural Sciences Courses at the University of Missouri-Columbia', *Academic Medicine*, 67(5): 349–50.

Vilkinas, T. and Cartan, G. (1990) 'A Preferred Approach to Management Education has a Learner-centred and Problem-based Emphasis', *Higher Education Research and Development*, 9(1): 71–9.

Walton, H. J. and Matthews, M. B. (1989) 'Essentials of Problem-based Learning', *Medical Education*, 23(6): 542–58.

Wilkerson, L. and Feletti, G. (1992) *Problem-Based Learning: One Approach to Increasing Student Participation in the Classroom*, Boston, Massachusetts: Harvard Medical School.

Wilkerson, L. and Maxwell, J. A. (1988) 'A Qualitative Study of Initial Faculty Tutors in a Problem-based Curriculum', *Journal of Medical Education*, 63: 892–9.

Wong, S. (1978) 'Nurse-teacher Behaviours in the Clinical Field: Apparent Effects on Nursing Students' Learning', *Journal of Advanced Nursing*, 3: 369–72.

Woods, D. R. (1985) 'What about Problem-based Learning?', *Journal of College Science Teaching*, Sept-Oct: 62–4.

Zerbe, M. and Luchat, M. (1991) 'A Three-Tiered Team Model for Undergraduate Preceptor Programmes', *Nurse Educator*, 16(2): 18–21.

Index